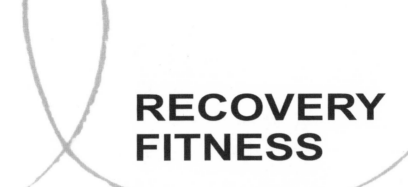

RECOVERY FITNESS

Exercises for Cancer Survivors

D1445330

Carol Michaels

and

Maria Drozda

Produced by:

FriesenPress

Suite 300 – 852 Fort Street
Victoria, BC, Canada V8W 1H8

www.friesenpress.com

Distributed to the trade by The Ingram Book Company

I dedicate this book to my parents, aunts, uncles, grandparents, friends and clients who have had cancer surgery and treatments. Their strength and courage provided the inspiration for the book.

It is my hope that your recovery from cancer surgery and treatments will be improved by performing the exercises in this book. I hope it will help you return to the things that you enjoyed prior to your diagnosis and improve your quality of life.

- Carol Michaels

I dedicate this book to my family members and friends who have battled cancer: those who have made excellent recoveries, those who continue to fight bravely and those who are now in heaven. Much strength, love and peace to you all.

- Maria Drozda

A portion of the profit from this book will be donated to cancer support and research charities. Increased funding for cancer research is desperately needed so that we can learn how to cure and ultimately prevent cancer.

Acknowledgements

Numerous people lent their expertise and experience to help create this book. Thank you to all of the health professionals at Morristown Medical Center and Barnabas Health for your support. A special thank you to Dr. and Mrs. Milton Michaels and Dr. Marian Michaels for your guidance and knowledge, which helped me create the Recovery Fitness® cancer exercise program.

I would like to express my gratitude to my clients and to the oncology health professionals who have helped me fine-tune this program. Thank you to my clients and friends who have faced the challenges of cancer. You have taught me so much and have enriched my life.

A special thank you to my husband Eric and my children, Jon and Laura, for their love, guidance and support.

- Carol Michaels

From a Healthcare Professional

Carol Michaels is an outstanding fitness trainer and has developed the Recovery Fitness® program, an exercise program that provides an invaluable tool to anyone who has been diagnosed with and is recovering from cancer.

I am a psychiatric nurse practitioner on the faculty at Morristown Medical Center. I have a private practice and specialize in the care of cancer patients. When I first learned of Carol's innovative recovery fitness program I was immediately impressed with its thoughtful design and I immediately started to refer patients to her. The feedback that I received from my patients was consistent: they were all delighted with the care she took with each of them and her obvious expertise at fitness training. They were equally pleased with how the program and Carol made them feel: good about themselves, more relaxed, calmer and simply better.

Not only is Carol excellent at what she does - helping patients regain and improve their physical strength and mobility - she is compassionate, thoughtful and dedicated. Moreover, the oncologists with whom I have worked have been extremely impressed with the progress their patients have made under Carol's care and we are all grateful to have her and her program as a resource.

The benefit to patients who participate in Carol's Recovery Fitness® program goes way beyond their physical fitness (which in and of itself is no small feat). Not only do my patients improve physically, but also they begin to feel better about themselves and more hopeful about the future. The stronger and more mobile that they become, the more they are able to imagine beating their cancer. This creates a positive cycle that fills them with hope and heals not only their external ailment but also their internal and psychological wounds.

Now Carol's extraordinary Recovery Fitness® program is available to everyone in book form. This is truly a road map back to fitness.

Randi Cohen, APN, BC
Family/Adult Psychiatric Nurse Practitioner

From a Recovery Fitness® Client

My name is Liz Johnson and I am a breast cancer conscript. Beating cancer is only part of the problem. Living with the body that's left after treatment for me was the greater challenge. My diagnosis called for chemotherapy, a double mastectomy and radiation. The surgery meant using chest muscles in new ways and shortening my lymphatic veins. Add radiation to the equation, and I was at high risk for developing infections, painfully tight muscles and skin and lymphedema - characterized by "elephant-sized" arms. Gratefully, I had doctors who recommended exercise throughout treatment.

That's where Carol Michaels came in. Her strength and stretch classes are constructed so that any student, regardless of fitness level or mobility issues, can get the help they need.

In my case, I took the classes as soon as I was able to after surgery and all through radiation. On days I took her class I could feel the difference - I had less tightness, soreness and swelling brought on by radiation. I also believe the classes helped me heal faster. I now have full range of motion in both arms and am able to return to the activities I enjoy such as swimming, biking and running.

Carol was great at customizing the exercises so that I worked the areas I needed to, but could also pull back so that I didn't overdo it, which is key when facing issues like lymphedema. I found her knowledge of physiology, anatomy and how cancer treatment affects them illuminating, helpful and a great comfort when facing the uncertainty of a cancer diagnosis. She's fabulous.

I highly recommend her program as outlined in this book to anyone going through cancer treatment or recovering from it. This book is an empowering guide for those that want to improve their quality of life after cancer.

Liz Johnson
Frenchtown, NJ

Contents

Foreword

Exercise is an important component of a cancer survivor's recovery process. Emerging research suggests a decrease in breast cancer recurrence for those who exercise. A well-designed program can also decrease side effects and improve quality of life. Moreover, acceptance of exercise as part of a good recuperation and standard of care has been gaining momentum in the medical community.

After surgery, I want my patients to begin an exercise program designed to ameliorate the adverse effects of surgery and help them regain their pre-cancer fitness level. Exercise that focuses on functional fitness will help them be able to perform the activities of daily living and return to the activities that they enjoy.

My patients, however, always have questions about exercise. Which exercises should I be doing and which should I avoid? Can I exercise during chemotherapy? Can I exercise if I have lymphedema? How do I exercise safely with osteoporosis? Some patients will need to exercise under supervision while others will be able to exercise independently. The type and scope of cancer and the overall medical condition and fitness level of a patient will determine whether or not a supervised program is needed. This book, *Recovery Fitness Exercises for Cancer Survivors*, will be an essential guide for those who prefer or need to exercise independently.

For those who do not live near a major city, it might be difficult to find a therapist who has experience working with cancer patients. This book provides cancer survivors with access to fitness tools specifically created for their needs. It can also be a valuable tool for those who cannot afford health care, or are unable to leave their house. Exercise is a simple and affordable treatment.

Carol Michaels is a cancer exercise specialist who knows how to customize a program that is right for her clients. She is able to create exercises and exercise programs based on each of her client's surgery, treatments, and fitness level. Carol has now taken her Recovery Fitness® exercise program and created this book to help you. You should use the exercises in this book as a guide to building an individualized routine that works and feels right for you.

This book will teach you how to prevent injury. Cancer survivors need to be patient; returning to your pre-cancer fitness level takes time and cannot be rushed. You will learn the implications of your particular surgery and the corrective exercises needed to improve recovery. *Recovery Fitness Exercises for Cancer Survivors* is a great way for cancer survivors to learn stretching and strength training exercise. My patients who participate in exercise programs say that it is empowering and gives them a sense of control and accomplishment.

Good luck!

Deborah Axelrod, MD, FACS

Clinical Director, Breast Services and Programs
Kanas Family Foundation Associate Professor of Surgery
NYU School of Medicine

Introduction

The importance of maintaining an active lifestyle and engaging in regular exercise has been emphasized more and more in recent years as the benefits for health, weight management and general well-being have been demonstrated in numerous studies.

At the same time, the number of persons in the United States with a history of cancer has continued to rise, and these individuals often face unique challenges with regard to exercise, either during their cancer treatment or in the months and years after their treatment is concluded.

During and after treatment for cancer, many survivors experience persistent fatigue, deficits in strength and range of motion, and decreased ability to manage the work and home tasks they previously enjoyed.

Exercise and fitness training have special benefits for patients during and after treatment for cancer. During chemotherapy, studies have indicated that exercise may increase fitness and energy levels, improve mood, and help patients better tolerate cancer treatments. After treatment is concluded, exercise can increase strength and aerobic capacity, improve joint flexibility, elevate mood, and assist with resumption of regular activities and work demands. In addition, exercise has been shown to decrease the risk of onset or recurrence of many types of cancer.

Individuals with or at risk for lymphedema after lymph node removal and/ or irradiation are a unique group, because for many years it was assumed that using the at-risk arm or leg for strenuous activities increased the risk of developing lymphedema, or worsened pre-existing lymphedema. Fortunately, studies over the last few years have shown these fears to be unfounded, and in fact have suggested that regular exercise, even strength training, may decrease the risk of lymphedema or diminish symptoms of lymphedema already present.

The program outlined in this book is intended to teach cancer survivors safe and correct exercises, with adaptations suggested for particular types of cancer and cancer treatments. Cancer survivors will learn how to perform exercises safely and using good technique to improve flexibility, strength and function. Slow progression of exercise is stressed while monitoring for fullness or aching that can indicate possible problems with lymphedema.

The exercises demonstrated, when used in conjunction with regular follow-up with an individual's medical team, are generally safe both for those at risk for lymphedema and those with lymphedema. Safety and appropriate precautions are emphasized throughout the book. One of the goals of *Recovery Fitness Exercises for Cancer Survivors* is to encourage fitness without incurring pain or injury that could trigger or exacerbate lymphedema. This book will help provide readers with the information they need to begin and continue a safe and effective exercise program during and after treatment for cancer so that they can enjoy the many physical and psychological benefits of exercise over the long term.

Kathleen Francis, MD

Medical Director, Barnabas Health ACC Lymphedema Treatment Center
Lymphedema Physician Services, P.C.

After breast cancer surgery, I advise my patients to take steps in a positive direction and improve their emotional, spiritual and physical health. Our physical bodies carry us through this life and are intimately connected to our emotional and spiritual health. We cannot heal one without the others. I personally have changed my life for the better by starting and maintaining a regular exercise program. Part of my responsibility as a healer is to inspire my patients to take care of their own bodies after breast cancer treatment.

Carol Michaels's sensitive and personal approach to cancer recovery fitness has helped so many of my patients achieve wholeness and the ability to be optimistic about life again. This is a vital part of the recovery process.

Nancy Elliott, MD, FACS
Director, Montclair Breast Center

Program Background

Cancer has been part of my world for over thirty years. My mother, father, and many other family members and friends have battled this disease. I have cared for and watched loved ones suffer and often die from this disease. As a result, one of my life goals was to do whatever I could to help the healing process. I needed to make an impact on a deep level. As a fitness professional, I worked with people of all ages and fitness levels. My career also brought me in contact with many people who were suffering from the side effects of cancer surgery and treatments. I then determined that I had to help these clients improve their quality of life through exercise, an essential component of the recovery process. This resulted in my creating the Recovery Fitness® cancer exercise program, which was inspired by and is dedicated to these courageous people.

A goal of many people recovering from surgery is to be able to return to the things that they enjoy. Cancer patients often have a difficult time recovering and develop frozen shoulder, stiffness, and numbness due to surgery and treatments. After surgery, it is important to build strength and flexibility in the chest, shoulder, abdomen, and back. Because many of these side effects can be prevented through proper exercise, I created a series of stretches and strengthening exercises to help eliminate or minimize these side effects.

Sometimes, patients are so overwhelmed by their diagnosis that they do not comprehend the specifics of the chemotherapy or the exact details of the surgery. Reconstructive surgery, such as TRAM flap (Transverse Rectus Abdominis Myocutaneous) and LAT flap (Latissimus Dorsi Tissue), changes muscle location. It is important to strengthen certain muscle groups that will have to compensate for the changes that have occurred during the surgery. My program helps to teach patients the very important tools of how to exercise properly and safely. Cancer survivors need these corrective exercises. It is imperative for them to reach a fitness level that provides confidence and peace of mind.

I have demonstrated that the Recovery Fitness® program is medically sound, and I have had internists, surgeons, and oncologists endorse the program. The value of adding a fitness professional to the patient's team is finally receiving the acknowledgment that it deserves by the medical community.

Program Description

The Recovery Fitness® cancer exercise program is a series of stretching and strengthening exercises designed to improve recovery. These exercises range from stretches done as you progress from being in bed, moving to a chair and finally to the point where you are able to lift light weights. The program shows you how to work out, when to work out, and the duration and frequency of the workouts. If you follow the Recovery Fitness® cancer exercise program, the difficult experience of having cancer can be made a lot easier. As you read through this book, you will notice that we repeat a lot of common themes. These will help to reinforce the underlying rationale for our exercises.

Recovery Fitness® offers comprehensive advice so that you can begin improving your physical and emotional health and reclaim your life beyond cancer. Through exercise, you will regain some control over your body, manage side effects more successfully, and increase your body's ability to heal.

This book gives you clear concise directions to safely start an exercise program, and the tools to make exercise a lasting part of your lifestyle. You don't need a gym to perform the exercises the book recommends; most homes will have everything you will need.

The Recovery Fitness® book uses easy-to-perform exercises with easy-to-read descriptions. The book is intended to assist patients currently battling the disease as well as those who have been in remission for years. The recommendations in the Recovery Fitness® program can help make you stronger, fitter, and mentally prepared to battle cancer.

Why do you need *Recovery Fitness Exercises for Cancer Survivors?*

- Hospital or clinic classes may be too far away
- Fitness centers may not be hygienic enough for your weakened immune system
- There may not be a suitable program in close proximity
- You may prefer to exercise in the privacy of your home
- You can select the time that is convenient for you
- You can exercise when you have less fatigue
- Using books and DVDs to exercise can save money
- You can vary your routine so that you don't get bored

When some people hear the word exercise, they might immediately think about a difficult gym class or boot camp. The exercises in this book are gentle, safe, and effective. They are not high intensity. Exercise might be the last thing on your mind after a cancer diagnosis. As thousands of cancer survivors are finding, a good fitness program will help you build up your strength, improve your mood and help your recovery.

Exercise should be part of your treatment plan because it may:

♦ Decrease body fat to help lower estrogen levels

♦ Reduce circulating testosterone

♦ Improve the immune system

♦ Decrease insulin levels

♦ Reduce pain from cancer treatments

Chapter 1

Exercising Safely

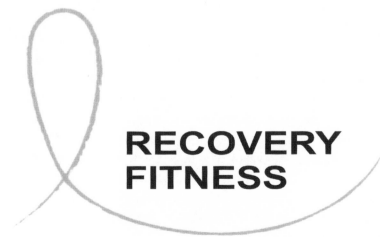

RECOVERY FITNESS

Exercising Safely

Exercise may be the furthest thing from your mind after a cancer diagnosis. Even if you have never been active, exercise can become one of your favorite activities. Ask your doctor before you start to exercise because each person is unique and heals differently. With more medical professionals recommending exercise to their patients, it is imperative for cancer survivors to learn how to exercise safely. A good exercise program will help to reduce the side effects of surgery and treatments. These side effects can include fatigue, neuropathy, decreased range of motion, weakness, lymphedema, and a significant emotional toll. Once you start to exercise and have less pain, stiffness and more energy, you will be motivated to continue. This book is an essential tool for the recovery process, especially for those who do not have access to a cancer exercise specialist, physical therapist, or are of limited means. Cancer can be a wake-up call for you to make healthy lifestyle changes.

Exercise may reduce the chance of recurrence, and it is therefore more important than ever to add exercise to your recovery plan. For those who have been active prior to their diagnosis, this is great news. The exercises described in this book will help to get you back to the activities that you enjoy. For the cancer survivors who are inactive, this book will give you the tools that you need to get started in an exercise program that is part of a healthy lifestyle.

Before You Begin

You will need to speak to your health professional before beginning the exercises contained in this book. Your particular surgery, treatments, fitness level and healing speed will guide the progression of the exercises. Your health and recovery process is always changing and it will be important to regularly monitor your blood count, muscle and joint pain, nausea, and fatigue. You may also have lingering impairments or health concerns that need to be evaluated by a physical therapist or lymphedema therapist.

You should meet with your oncologist to review the exact nature of your treatments so that you will understand the potential side effects of your treatments. This way you will be able to understand your exercise plan in relation to your unique situation. For example, Arimedex may make your joints or muscles sore. Some medications affect balance and cardiac function, or increase the risk of dehydration. It is crucial that you understand the health issues you may encounter as a consequence of your surgery or treatment. This will include learning which muscles are affected, which lymph nodes are removed, and the cardiac and pulmonary effects of radiation and chemotherapy.

Exercise Goals

Goals should be specific and realistic. You may want to lose weight and increase your muscle mass. If flexibility is an issue, your goal may be to improve your range of motion. Other goals might be to become stronger, have a good quality of life, better mood, or to decrease the chance of recurrence.

It is helpful to have both short term and long term exercise goals. Goals should be able to be adapted to changes in work, health, and family situations. If you are new to exercise, select an activity and set an achievable goal. Slowly add exercise to your daily activities and find something that works with your lifestyle.

Remember: Think positive and have fun!

Exercising During Chemotherapy and Radiation

It seems counterintuitive, but exercise during treatment is shown to be helpful. Physical activity during treatment can reduce common side effects such as fatigue, pain, nausea, depression or anxiety. If you are suffering from pain and nausea you should have those issues under control before beginning. Your doctor will be able to tell you how often you should exercise and how intense your program should be.

Each treatment has unique and has potentially debilitating side effects of which you should be aware.

Systemic treatments such as chemotherapy and hormonal therapy as well as targeted, biological and immunotherapies may impact your balance, cardiac function, and gastro-intestinal tract. Furthermore, they may lead to neuropathy or numbness in your extremities.

Breast cancer patients are often on hormonal therapy. Common medications such as aromatase inhibitors (post-menopause) and Tamoxifen can lead to weight gain, joint pain, muscle pain, and other menopause-related symptoms including bone density loss. Other treatments for breast cancer, such as Herceptin, may have side effects that need to be reviewed with your doctor.

Radiation can cause fatigue and increases the risk of lymphedema. It can also cause swelling and burning of the skin.

First Steps

Try to start moving as soon as possible after surgery, even if it is only walking indoors. This will help you to regain strength. Although only one limb may be affected by your surgery, try to move both limbs equally. If you had been inactive prior to surgery, start with short walks and increase the distance walked each time. You can also increase the frequency of the walks as you slowly increase the distance. Try to find a walking buddy and walk often. Build up strength slowly and make sure never to over do it. Just 15 minutes a day can improve your energy level and mood.

Although this book focuses on stretching and strengthening, we recommend that you incorporate aerobic activity in your fitness plan. Find the aerobic activity – one that increases your heart and breathing rate – that you enjoy and try to do it daily. Aerobic activity is an important component of a fitness plan and includes activities like walking, hiking, and dancing.

Precautions for Stretching and Strengthening

1. Your immune system may be compromised, which places you at risk for infection. Gyms carry a high risk for infection. One of my motivating factors for writing this book was to help patients to be able to exercise at home while their immune system is weak.

2. If you have poor balance, you may want to start with the exercises that are safer for those who have balance problems. Poor balance may be due to the chemotherapy, weak muscles, neurological issues, or normal aging. A common side effect of chemotherapy is peripheral neuropathy, which changes the sensation in the legs or arms. It can last a short time or be long lasting. This can affect the way you walk, your balance, and your general movement. If you have peripheral neuropathy, you should select activities that decrease your risk of falling. For example, we recommend avoiding uneven surfaces and exercising with a stationary bike instead of a treadmill without handles. Strengthening your core will help your balance. It is also a good idea to keep all the muscles strong to compensate for the ones that are affected by the neuropathy.

3. Be smart and safe by doing the exercises that are right for you at this particular time. You are exercising to get healthy, not to get hurt. This is an important point to keep in mind, particularly for those who were physically active before cancer. You will not be able to immediately resume the same level of pre-cancer activity.

4. Exercise in a temperature controlled environment. Cold temperature can crack your skin, while extreme heat can cause swelling or light-headedness.

5. At the start of your exercise program, you should warm up with deep breathing techniques and shoulder rolls. We recommend that you warm up before you stretch by walking, marching in place or using a stationary bike. You can also exercise after a warm shower, which may relax the muscles.

6. Never hold your breath during an activity. People often hold their breath during exercise, so remember to breathe deeply.

7. Drink plenty of water, especially when sweating.

8. If your blood counts or the mineral levels (potassium and sodium) are low, check with your health professional before resuming exercise.

9. Some medications affect the heart rate, so your pulse rate is not a good indicator of the level of your exercise exertion.

10. Learn to move slowly and smoothly without jerky movements. Do not continue an activity if it causes pain or unusual fatigue. You should feel a gentle stretch, not pain.

11. Know your limits. You should be able to differentiate between discomfort and unusual pain. Stop if you feel pain. Listen to your body and use common sense. If something does not feel right, do not do it. You should consult with your doctor if you are experiencing pain, swelling, or unusual fatigue.

12. Wear comfortable and loose clothing and appropriate footwear. For those with peripheral neuropathy affecting the feet, supportive footwear is particularly important.

Precautions for Strength Training

1. Add strength training after you have achieved almost full range of motion. You do not want to be stronger in a limited plane of motion. If you are able to touch your opposite ear by placing your arm over your head without feeling a stretch, you can start to slowly add strength training exercises. If you take a few days off from exercising, decrease the amount of weight used when you return to strength training.

2. We recommend that you warm up before strength training by walking, marching in place, or using a stationary bike.

3. Good form is important. Focus on quality over quantity of repetitions.

4. Rotate your muscle groups so that you don't overwork the muscles in one area.

5. Avoid the natural tendency to use heavier weights on your stronger side. Your weaker side will set the limits on the amount of weight used. This is determined by the amount of weight that you can lift for 10 repetitions in perfect form, feeling some fatigue by the eighth repetition.

6. Aim for slow gradual improvement and gradually increase the weight that you use. We suggest that you increase the amount of weight used in 1-pound increments. Having patience will prevent you from using a heavy weight and causing a problem. Being patient and consistent will help you achieve your goals. *Remember: quality over quantity.*

7. Wait 48 hours between strength training sessions. Use the day in between strength training sessions for aerobic exercise and stretching.

8. Cool down after you exercise by walking or stretching,

9. Understand your lymphedema risk. Although lymphedema may not be evident, your lymphatic system may function below normal. The National Lymphedema Network recommends that at-risk individuals wear a well-fitted compression garment while exercising their affected limb. A gradual, progressive strength-training program may actually minimize the chance of developing lymphedema by widening the remaining lymphatic channels. Wide channels can handle the increase in the flow of lymph created by vigorous exercise. Stretches can ease tightness and scarring that block lymphatic flow. Lymphedema is discussed in greater detail in Chapter 9.

Chapter 2

When, Why and How to Start

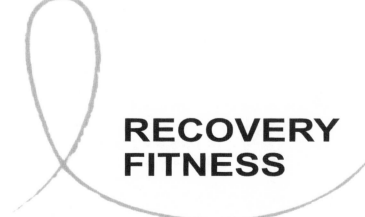

RECOVERY FITNESS

Cancer surgery and treatments affect many areas of the body. I hear numerous complaints of stiffness, pulling, tightness, and a lack of flexibility. Often this occurs when the muscles and skin are shortened because of the surgery, which can also leave scar tissue. Surgery can irritate the nerves. As a result, you may feel burning, tingling, or numbness.

When to Start

When can you start an exercise program after having cancer surgery and treatments? You should start stretching exercises as soon as you get clearance from your doctor. It is important to talk to your doctor before starting to exercise. This way you can determine what program is right for you. Some exercises can be started soon after surgery while others can be done right after the drains and stitches are removed.

For those who have access to post-surgery specialists, at the start of your exercise program for breast cancer, a physical therapist or cancer exercise specialist takes range of motion measurements of the shoulder. These include shoulder flexion, extension, abduction and rotation measurements. For example, you may start with only 30 degrees of shoulder flexion and after several months reach significant improvement. My clients have improved shoulder flexion by over 140 degrees over periods ranging from two weeks to three months. Everyone heals at a different rate. In an ideal situation it is helpful to take these measurements prior to the surgery. This gives you a basis of comparison.

It is also a good idea to meet with a lymphedema therapist if you are at risk for lymphedema. This way the lymphedema therapist can take limb girth measurements. These can be used a basis of comparison if there is suspicion of lymphedema.

Why and How to Start

Emotional Health

Exercise is good for our emotional health. It is one thing that you can control and do for yourself. It is empowering. Physical activity can decrease depression and anxiety. Participants in my program reduce stress, increase confidence and build positive health habits. The participants also gain endurance, increase their energy level and decrease the fatigue that may be caused by treatments.

Exercise Progression

Many variables determine the exercises that are effective and safe for your particular situation. Every day brings new challenges and new accomplishments for the cancer patient. It is important to be able to modify your exercises to fit your needs at a given time.

Pain and fatigue levels can change from day to day, and even from hour to hour. You may wake up feeling fine, but may have increased fatigue as the day progresses. Track your energy levels throughout the day to determine the best time to schedule your exercise sessions. For example, if you have more energy in the afternoons, you should exercise in the afternoons.

Use this book when your energy levels are high. Common sense and listening to your body are of utmost importance. You should not feel like you have to follow a set protocol or a strict schedule. Your routine must be customized due to the numerous physical and psychological side effects you may be experiencing.

Both healing times and pain tolerance can differ greatly from one person to the next. Speed of recovery depends on your pre-surgery fitness level and type of surgery and treatments. The progression and timing of a cancer exercise program can only be determined after a thorough discussion between the patient and her or his healthcare professional.

Relaxation Breathing

There is an emotional toll that cancer survivors face in addition to the physical one. A cancer diagnosis can cause depression, anger, anxiety, fear and stress. Proper breathing techniques and stretching can improve the psychological recovery.

For example, research has shown that breathing can help reduce stress and anxiety. When feeling stressed, we usually take shallow breaths. During these exercises we will use our full lung capacity and breathe slowly and deeply. You should be aware of your breathing as it has a calming effect. Inhale for 5 seconds and fill the torso up with air, then exhale from the lower abdomen for 5 seconds, pressing the navel in towards the spine. Imagine all of your tension and stress leaving your body with each exhalation.

You should begin relaxation breathing immediately after surgery, as it allows you to focus all your energy on healing. The stretching program will restore mobility in the chest and back that allows for freer movement of the lungs and diaphragm.

Aerobic Exercise

Aerobic exercise is essential for good health. This includes any movement that elevates your heart rate. As soon as you have medical clearance, you should start walking. Chemotherapy and radiation can cause fatigue. It may seem counterintuitive, but physical activity can help decrease fatigue and help you improve your ability to tolerate treatments. Walking can boost your energy. You might be able to walk only one house distance at first. Every day, try to walk farther until you are able to walk for 30-45 minutes. If this is not possible because of your health issues, aim for 15 minutes one to three times a day. Try to exercise when you feel the least tired. You may feel exhausted at various times during treatment and recovery, especially during chemotherapy or radiation. When you feel better, try to do more. Ultimately, the workout will help energize you and ease aches and pains.

Stretching

Stretching should be performed every day for a year or longer depending on your particular situation. And the older you are, the more important daily stretching is to maintain flexibility. Commit to stretching regularly so that you gradually improve your posture, range of motion, and flexibility.

First, warm up for 5-10 minutes by marching in place or use a stationary bicycle while swinging your arms. Then perform the stretching exercises 2-5 times per day in the beginning of your recovery. Use only smooth, controlled non-bouncy movements.

All movements should be done slowly and with great concentration. Try to reach the maximum pain-free range of motion possible for you. Do the stretches slowly and allow the tissue to lengthen. Hold the stretch until you feel a little tension, but not to the point of pain. The goals are to restore joint mobility and break down residual scar tissue. If you can't stretch as shown in the photograph, modify the stretch to your ability by only going a fraction of the distance.

At first, you might suffer from fatigue and low endurance and might only be able to exercise for a short period of time. Every day you can lengthen the session. Patience and practice will pay off. As you get stronger, you can increase the length of your sessions.

Once you have achieved an acceptable range of motion, it is usually necessary to continue your stretching program so you can maintain that range of motion. If you have had radiation, stretching is very important to help keep your body flexible. Radiation typically causes additional tightening. Radiation can impact the affected area for a year or longer after the treatment is finished.

Important!
If you notice swelling or tenderness, contact your health professional.

Strength Training

Next up is strength training. Strength training improves balance and posture by improving core strength. It can improve your quality of life by making activities easier and more enjoyable. It can also reduce the chance of injury and can empower you physically and mentally.

Another reason to strength train is that chemotherapy can cause weight gain and can change the muscle-to-fat ratio. Strength training improves the muscle-to-fat ratio. We need to gain muscle mass, which can decrease during treatments, and we need to strengthen bones. Having more muscle will increase metabolism. A pound of muscle burns twice as many calories as does a pound of fat. So strength training is a great way to help get to or keep your weight at a healthy level. While diet is often the most critical factor for weight loss, and is beyond the scope of this book, strength training is a major factor as well.

Many cancer treatments can increase the risk for osteoporosis. Strength training helps build strong bones. You need to learn which exercises are contraindicated for osteoporosis. For example, if you have or are at risk for osteoporosis you should not do forward bends, abdominal crunches or extreme twisting movements. See Chapter 8 for more information on osteoporosis.

Surgery can lead to weakness in your muscles in the chest, shoulders, abdomen or back. We need to rebuild strength in the areas affected and keep all the muscles in the body strong, as well as correct muscle imbalances.

After you have achieved an acceptable range of motion, posture, and have medical clearance, it will be time to add strength training. Exercise gently, focusing on slow and progressive improvement. Control and good form are essential.

Chapter 3

Mindful Stretching

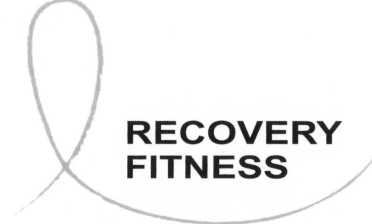

RECOVERY FITNESS

Mindful Stretching

Stretching is one of the basic components of fitness. The goal from stretching is to improve your range of motion, which is the degree of movement that can be achieved without pain. Elongating the muscle and fascia by stretching improves circulation, increases elasticity of the muscle, increases oxygen to the muscles, and helps the body to repair.

The Recovery Fitness® program uses a combination of active stretching and static stretching.

In active or dynamic stretching, the stretch is held for 1-2 seconds and repeated 10 times. In static stretching, the stretch is maintained for approximately 10-30 seconds and can be repeated several (2-3) times. You should move in and out of each stretch slowly and smoothly.

An active stretch helps muscles relax. An example is shoulder flexion:

Bring the arm upward and hold for 1-2 seconds and then lower it back to your starting position. Repeat 10 times. With each repetition, raise the arm higher until you feel tension, but not pain. Exhale as you bring your arm up and inhale as you bring your arm down. 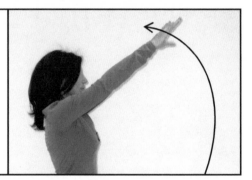

Active stretching is used in the beginning of your session. After you are warmed up, you can begin to hold the stretch longer and alternate between static and active stretching. Our muscles work in pairs: one muscle works or contracts, while the other relaxes or lengthens. As your stretching session progresses you will determine how long to hold the stretch. The amount of time one should hold a stretch depends on the individual. By listening to your body and using common sense, you will be able to determine what feels good and what works best.

Effective Stretching

♦ Before stretching, you should warm up. Stretching is more effective when warm, as your muscles and tendons are easier to lengthen.

- The brain and nervous system work together in every stretch, and every repetition causes neuromuscular education. By thinking about the movement and concentrating on the affected muscle, we rewire the injured or tight muscle. Be mindful of the movement and its purpose.

- Slowly lengthen the muscle to a comfortable length while using relaxation breathing (see page 20).

- The stretches should feel good. Hold the stretch until you feel tension. As you hold the stretch the muscle will relax and you will be able to increase the stretch. Each day it will get easier and you will see your flexibility improve.

- Modify the stretches to take in to account your day-to-day pain and fatigue levels. Do not worry if you are less flexible on a particular day. Just do your best and modify the stretch as needed. You might only be able to perform a few of the stretches on a particular day, or you may need to decrease the length of your session. You may also modify your flexibility routine by reducing the amount of time the stretch is held or changing the number of repetitions performed.

- The stretches in this book can be performed while standing, sitting, or lying on the floor. Most can even be done in bed. If you feel mild pain, place a small pillow under your head or anywhere that reduces it.

- The stretches in this book can be performed in several ways. Add a variety of angles to each stretch. For example, if you perform a shoulder stretch with your arm parallel to the floor, try doing the same stretch with the arm at an angle pointing toward the ceiling.

Why should you continue to stretch even after achieving full range of motion?

- Stretching improves flexibility, which is the range of motion at a joint or group of joints. It increases the circulation of blood to the muscles and prevents tight muscles, which have less blood flow. The blood carries oxygen that the muscle needs for energy. Blood flow also removes lactic acid and carbon dioxide, which cause inflammation.

  Stretching, especially active or dynamic stretching, helps you to get ready for any physical activity. Examples of dynamic stretches are walking lunges, squats, and arm circles. Dynamic stretching acts as a warm-up to reduce injuries, get the muscles warm, and improve performance. Being flexible helps generate speed and power.

♦ Stretching improves posture. See Chapter 5 for more information on posture.

♦ Each movement helps to move lymph through the body.

♦ Stretching improves movement patterns and decreases the chance of developing over-use injuries.

♦ Stretching with relaxation breathing reduces stress.

♦ Stretching increases feelings of well-being because you are able to perform your daily activities more easily and with less pain.

♦ Radiation treatment can cause additional tightening. Ongoing flexibility exercises are always recommended to those who have had radiation so that they are able to maintain their range of motion and all of the benefits that good flexibility brings.

Chapter 4

Strength Training

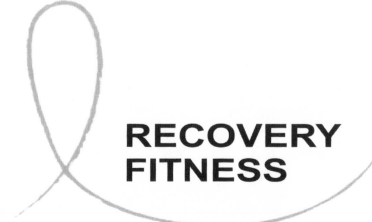

RECOVERY FITNESS

Strength Training

Strength training is the last phase of the Recovery Fitness® program. Strength training or resistance training is exercise using weights (or your own body weight) to strengthen and build muscle. It increases the size and strength of the muscle fibers and strengthens the tendons, ligaments, and bones.

Role of Muscles

It is important that you understand the role of your skeletal muscles. They move and support your skeleton and link two bones across their connecting joints. The skeletal muscles work with your bones to give your body power and strength. When these muscles contract or shorten, your bone moves. Muscles that move bones act together in pairs. This means that as one muscle contracts, its partner relaxes. Then as the partner muscle contracts, the first muscle relaxes again.

Benefits of Strength Training

It is necessary to strength train because we lose muscle mass as we age. This loss of muscle may be compounded by your treatments. The good news is that you can reverse this muscle loss at any age. Muscles are metabolically active. This means that they burn calories at rest and during exercise. Strength training helps to increase our muscle mass. Since muscle is metabolically active, more muscle mass means a faster metabolism. Therefore, strength training can help you keep your weight under control and help with weight loss. This is especially important to cancer survivors because the treatments can cause weight gain.

Strength or resistance training can also decrease your risk of injury and improve athletic performance. It improves balance, agility, coordination, and energy levels at all ages.

This book uses gentle strength training techniques:

♦ If an exercise hurts, decrease the weight or do not do that particular exercise.

♦ Do not ever push through pain. If it hurts, you're overdoing it and could be injured.

♦ Use a light weight or light resistance bands. A 1-2 pound can of food works.

♦ Exercise in front of a mirror to watch your form.

♦ Keep your back flat with the abs contracted to support the lower back.

Weights

Strength training can be performed using free weights, resistance bands or machines. Free weights (also known as dumbbells or hand weights) are used in this program. Ideally, you should have a variety of free weights ranging from 1-5 pounds. Resistance bands are good for strength training at work or while travelling. It can be difficult, however, to measure the amount of tension used. If you use resistance bands and are at risk for lymphedema, you should not grip the band tightly or wrap it around your hand.

I am often asked by clients whether they should use machines or free weights. Although machines can be helpful for those who have problems with balance, exercise with free weights has several benefits. First, they allow you to strength train at home at your convenience and you can improve by 1-pound increments. Using free weights allows you to strengthen more major muscle groups without depending on a machine for support. Weight machines work only the large muscle groups. They can miss the small, but important stabilizer muscles, which help with balance, coordination and injury prevention.

Frequency

A 'repetition' (rep) is one complete motion of an exercise. A 'set' is a group of consecutive repetitions. In this program, one set consists of 5-10 reps. You should try to strength train twice a week. Strengthen each muscle group, alternating from upper to lower body. It is fine to rest between sets so you have strength to do the next exercise using perfect form. Work the front, back, and side of the body so that you do not create imbalances.

What weight should I use?

If you are new to exercise, you might start with no weight or with 1 pound. By the 5th to 8th rep you should feel the muscle working. By the 10th rep you should feel that you have worked the muscle, but are not exhausted. If you are exhausted, decrease the weight. To improve your strength, you will need to increase the weight you use. By slowly using more weight, you will increase muscle mass and strength. You want to get the most out of your exercise session, but not become injured. Do not increase the weight if it means sacrificing good form. Breathe during the exercise – exhale on the exertion (the lifting phase). Lift slowly and concentrate on controlling the weight on the way up and on the way down.

Remember: If you feel like you have not done anything, it's time to increase the weight.

Chapter 5

Posture

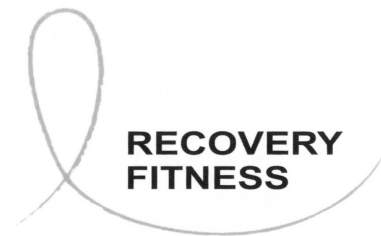

RECOVERY FITNESS

Posture

Good posture allows for efficient movement and is important for overall health. Poor posture can cause some muscles to work too hard and others too little. This causes physical imbalance and can result in some muscles becoming very weak and some too tight. Eventually joints can become stressed, which can lead to pain and poor range of motion. If you've ever had your back "go out", you know exactly what this means.

There are significant benefits to having good posture. These include efficient movement, improved strength, balance, and a decreased chance of muscle strain, tendonitis or bursitis. Proper posture will allow you to move with more freedom and make you feel more confident.

Poor posture can create muscle tightness and shortening which can also press on nerves, causing pain. Some back and neck discomfort can be alleviated through posture improvement. Many years ago, a physical therapist told me that half of his business is attributable to his clients having posture dysfunction. Some posture issues should be addressed by a physical therapist, posture specialist, or doctor.

As we age, it's common for the shoulders to round and for us to develop a head forward position. When one has a head forward position, the affected vertebrae can harm the discs and compress the surrounding nerves. The vertebrae need to be properly aligned; when posture is improved, there will be less compression on the nerves and decreased pain.

As desk jobs increase, the number of people with good posture decreases. Poor posture is now developing at younger and younger ages and is being observed even in our middle school population. This is partially due to the prevalence of hand-held devices, causing one to jut the head forward to read the screen, and to the amount of time spent sitting in front of a computer. Using the computer all day will lead to a rounding of a person's back and cause their chin to go forward. The way we position ourselves at our desks or on our sofas can also lead to poor posture and imbalances. This will lead to kyphosis at an early age. In kyphosis, one has a forward head, tight pectoral muscles and weak back muscles.

Even if you work on your stretches and strengthening exercises several times a week, you need to think about maintaining good posture every day. It's also a good idea to use proper ergonomics. Try not to carry a heavy bag on one side and make sure that your desk and chair are the right height for you. Stretch regularly throughout the day. Always think about sitting and standing up tall with your shoulders down and back.

Cancer Surgery and Treatments can Affect Posture

Studies have shown that if you have breast cancer surgery and treatments, you are more likely to develop faulty body posture. If you are having posture problems after surgery, you need to tell your health team.

After surgery, cancer survivors have a tendency to protect the area where they had the surgery. The chest area can feel tight and the cancer survivor compensates by rounding her shoulders. Muscles are shortened because of the surgery and there is scar tissue. Nerves may be irritated, which can result in numbness and tingling. It is important for you to learn the essential stretches for the pectoral muscles and shoulders. Eventually, you will incorporate strength training with an emphasis on strengthening your upper back muscles. This will help decrease the chance of developing round shoulders with a forward head posture.

Some of the reconstruction processes also change muscle placement, which may affect the posture of a cancer survivor. Whenever there is a change in muscle placement, it is advisable to have a postural assessment. Also, abdominal surgery can result in abdominal tightness, which in turn creates an initial tendency to walk leaning forward. The good news is that most posture issues due to surgery and treatments are easily corrected with proper stretching and strengthening exercises.

Posture Assessments

Performed by your Health or Fitness Professional

If it is available and you can afford it, you should have a monthly posture assessment in both a standing position and during physical activity. I recommend that you have a baseline posture assessment prior to surgery as a basis of comparison. I have found that the best way to conduct the standing assessment is to stand against the wall and be assessed from a front, back, and side view. For the evaluation, clothing needs to be form fitting. The head, upper back and buttocks should touch the wall.

I observe the head placement. Is the ear in line with the shoulder? The shoulder blades should lie flat without winging, and the shoulder should be over the hip. The ribcage should be over the pelvis and the chest should be open. The front of the hip bones should be over the pubic bones. The hips should be over the ankle joint and the knees should not be hyper-extended or flexed.

Is there a lot of space between the head and the wall? If so, that is head forward posture. Head forward posture or *kyphosis* is where the upper back curves forward. This usually goes hand in hand with a weak upper back, especially around the scapula. The pectoral muscles are usually tight in this condition.

Is there a lot of space between the lower back and the wall? This is *lordosis*, where the lower back curves too much. Strengthening the core can help to prevent it, as will stretching the hip flexors.

The posture stretches and strengthening exercises in this book can help you prevent posture problems and improve existing conditions. Once problems are detected, an exercise program with the goal of correcting imbalances should be started. The right strengthening of weak muscles and stretching of tight muscles can help prevent pain due to poor posture. It can also help improve balance and prevent injuries.

Many exercises in this book can improve posture.

Stretching

Exercise	Page	Exercise	Page
Neck Rotation	75	Twisting Pectoral Stretch	84
Lateral Neck Stretch	75	VW Stretch	85
Double Chin	76	Standing Cat Stretch	85
Shoulder Shrug	76	Arm Circles	87
Backward Shoulder Roll	76	Pectoral & Shoulder Stretch	89
Scapular Retraction	77	Butterfly Arms	106
Serratus Reach	77	Shoulder Opener	107
Posterior Shoulder Stretch	78	Torso Stretch	107
Shoulder Extension & Variations	81	Supine Rotator Cuff Stretch	108
The Scapular Clock	83	Floor Stretches with Roller	113
Pectoral Wall Stretch	84	Stretches with the Ball	115

Strengthening

Exercise	Page
Superman Exercises	122
Bent Over Row	135
Reverse Fly	135
Seated and Standing Row	139
Rotator Cuff	140
Lat Pull Down	140
Shoulder Exercise on the Ball	143

Chapter 6

Balance

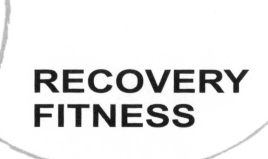

RECOVERY FITNESS

Balance

Falls and fall-related injuries, such as a hip fracture, can have serious consequences. If you fall, it could limit your activities or make it impossible to live independently. Balance and strength exercises can help prevent falls by improving your ability to control and maintain your body's position whether you are in motion or stationary.

Balance exercises will help you regain function and mobility for activities of daily living and are a key component for recovery after cancer treatments. Stability exercises can help to enhance both steadiness and leg strength. Balance training will help decrease the likeliness of falling.

Falls are dangerous for older women with weaker bones and for cancer survivors. Cancer survivors are at high risk for osteoporosis due to chemotherapy and cancer medications. If you are nervous about falling, you might withdraw from your daily activities and decrease your quality of life.

Surgery and Treatment Can Affect Your Balance

Your balance can suffer after surgical procedures. This is especially acute with the TRAM flap procedure where the *rectus abdominus* is altered. Poor core strength, caused by the change in placement of the *rectus abdominus*, has a negative effect on your balance. After a TRAM flap operation, you will need to learn how to compensate for this change of muscle placement through a series of exercises designed to strengthen the remaining muscles such as the obliques. Balance exercises can counter some of the effects of muscle imbalances and body asymmetry after surgery. Some of the chemotherapies can affect your balance. Neuropathy, which can make your feet numb, is a common side effect of chemotherapy. If you cannot feel your feet, it becomes difficult to maintain good balance. You should incorporate balance exercises as a regular part of your fitness routine.

The following exercises are aimed at improving your balance and your lower body strength. Start by holding on to a sturdy chair for support. To challenge yourself, start by holding the chair with only one hand. As you improve you will progress to holding the chair with only one finger and eventually you will be able to perform the exercise without holding the chair. To experience the importance of vision in balance, try some of the balance exercises with your eyes closed.

Balance exercises overlap with lower body strength exercises. Do the strength exercises that most relate to balance two or more days per week, but not on any two days in a row.

Start your balance exercise routine with the following eight exercises:

1. Standing on One Foot: hold for 10 seconds then switch legs

2. Tightrope: put your heel in front of the toe of the other foot walking a narrow path (put one foot in front of the other as if walking a tightrope)

3. Calf Raises (page 129) or Heel Raises: stand in place and raise each heel up and down

4. Front, Back, and Side Leg Lifts or Raises (pages 131-132)

5. Single Leg Stands: stand on one leg for 60 seconds then switch legs

6. Grapevines: step sideways while crossing one foot in front, and then in back of the other

7. Pelvic Tilt (page 119); beginning level core strength

8. Bridge (page 120); core and lower body strength

Many Exercises in this Book Can Improve Balance

Exercise	Page
Tai Chi Inspired Stretch	97
Standing Hip Stretch	99
Waitress Stretch	100
Weight Shift	102
Stretches with the Ball	115-116
Superman Exercises	122
Birddog and Variations	123-124
All Core Exercises	119-128
Wall Sit	129
Squats	133
Lunge	134
Strengthening Exercises with the Ball	141-143

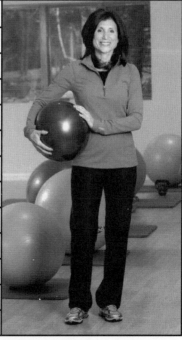

Chapter 7

Side Effects of Cancer Surgery and Treatments

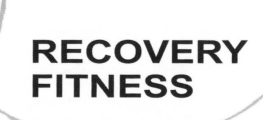

RECOVERY FITNESS

Side Effects of Cancer Surgery and Treatments

Surgery, chemotherapy, radiation, and hormonal therapy have side effects, which exacerbate the problems faced by cancer patients. Surgery can create adhesions that can limit range of motion, and cause pain, numbness and tightness. Removal of lymph nodes creates scars and may decrease range of motion. Chemotherapy may affect balance, a patient's immune system, and cause nausea, light-headedness, vertigo, neuropathy, fatigue, sarcopenia (loss of muscle mass), and anemia. Radiation can cause fatigue, tightness and stiffness. Surgery, chemotherapy and radiation can also increase the risk of developing lymphedema. Hormonal therapy can cause joint pain and early menopause and the side effects associated with menopause.

Cancer surgery and treatments affect the entire body, not just the area of the cancer. Everyone has different reactions to the treatments. Sometimes the effects become apparent after the treatment is finished. Some symptoms can appear years later, particularly lymphedema.

We will now discuss some of the side effects and the precautions you should take related to exercise. This will help you understand the issues and modifications needed to exercise safely. By understanding the potential side effects, you will know what to be mindful of and when to decrease exercise frequency and intensity.

Exercise Precautions for Fatigue

Cancer-related fatigue is the type of fatigue that does not leave even after resting. It may deter you from embarking on an exercise program. If you feel lethargic, decrease the intensity of the exercise. The following are some tips to help you overcome and exercise safely even when fatigued:

♦ Try to walk, even around the house.
♦ Perform breathing, stretching, and balance exercises on the high fatigue days.
♦ Exercise with a friend. A buddy can help motivate you.
♦ Listen to music.
♦ Break up your exercise session into smaller sessions.
♦ Schedule sessions when you have the most energy.
♦ Change your exercise routine so that you do not get bored.

- Keep a journal.
- Understand your limitations. Listen to your body.
- Progress at your own pace.
- Use common sense. Know when to rest.
- Exercise to tolerance.
- Stay hydrated. Drink before, during and after exercise.

Exercise Precautions for a Weak Immune System

If you are receiving or recently completed chemotherapy, your immune system will be weakened. It is important to avoid infections. Stay away from crowded places and places that are not cleaned regularly. Wash your hands often and call your doctor if you have a fever. This book will enable you to exercise at home and avoid infection.

Exercise Precautions for Neuropathy

Neuropathy is a common side effect of cancer surgery and treatment that affects the nervous system. Chemotherapy may damage the nerves in your arms or legs. When the neuropathy is in the hands or feet it is called 'peripheral neuropathy'. This causes numbness, loss of sensation, tingling and pain. If your hands are affected, it may be difficult to safely hold on to hand weights. Using tubing or resistance bands with handles is safer.

Balance training is advised for peripheral neuropathy affecting the toes and feet. Your balance might be affected because of the loss of feeling in the feet. You need to modify exercises so that you don't fall. You should not perform exercises that require a high level of balance.

Exercise Precautions for Myelosuppression

Treatments can affect bone marrow activity. Red and white blood cells and platelets are produced in the bone narrow. Treatment may cause you to have less platelets, so you might bruise or bleed easily. Use caution with machines and equipment.

Exercise Precautions for Neutropenia and Anemia

Neutropenia, which is a decrease in white blood cells, may develop. A decrease in white blood cells can increase your risk of infection. Stay away from crowds and unsanitary spaces.

Anemia can develop, which is a decrease in red blood cells. This will cause fatigue. Adapt your exercises to suit your energy level.

Exercise Precautions for Osteoporosis

Osteoporosis, a decrease in bone density, is a common side effect of treatments. See Chapter 8 for detailed information on osteoporosis.

Exercise Precautions for Bone Metastases

When cancer cells are lodged in the bone, there is a high risk of breaking a bone. Swimming and riding a stationary bike are safe exercises. Perform balance exercises and exercises that have a low risk of falling. Follow the same precautions as for osteoporosis, as outlined in Chapter 8.

Exercise Precautions for Cardiopulmonary Issues

Some treatments affect the heart. An exercise program for someone who has weak heart muscles or an irregular heart beat should begin under supervision. Your heart rate, blood pressure and breathing will need to be monitored. If you have clearance from your doctor, be conservative and exercise at low intensities.

Exercise Precautions for Lymphedema

As described previously, lymphedema is a swelling of the limb or trunk. It is a common side effect that can occur after the removal of lymph nodes. If you have or are at risk for lymphedema, you need, if at all possible, to be evaluated by a lymphedema specialist before you begin an exercise program. Exercise is encouraged if you have lymphedema, but you should consider using a compression garment. Maintaining your range of motion and avoiding infection are important. You may have to make some modifications to your exercise routine. Start slowly and improve slowly. If you notice swelling, see your doctor. See Chapter 9 for detailed information on lymphedema.

Chapter 8

Osteoporosis

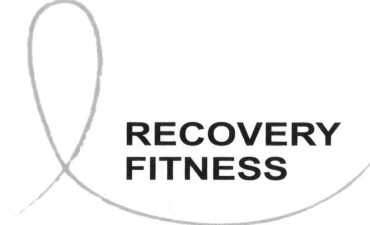

**RECOVERY
FITNESS**

Osteoporosis

Osteoporosis means porous bone and is a chronic disease that weakens the bones. It is a serious health issue. With osteoporosis, bone density decreases and the bones become fragile and break easily. Although it can cause a break in any bone, the most common sites for breaks are the hips, spine and wrist. A broken hip or spine usually requires a hospital stay or surgery and can lead to permanent pain, disability, or death.

Bone is Constantly Renewed Throughout our Lives

Our bodies are always breaking down bone and replacing it with new bone. In the re-absorption stage, the old bone is broken down and in the formation stage, new bone is built. As we age, the replacement process slows down. This causes the creation of bone-forming cells to begin to slow, which results in bone being lost at a faster pace than it is formed. The small spaces in the bone get larger as we lose bone density and the outside of the bone thins. Osteoporosis occurs as a result of an acceleration of this process, called primary osteoporosis. Secondary osteoporosis is caused by some medications and disease processes.

There Are No Symptoms in the Early Stages

Osteoporosis is a silent disease because it progresses without symptoms. Most people do not know that they have it until a bone breaks. The break can be the result of a fall or from something as slight as a bear hug. A sneeze or sudden movement can be enough to break a bone in someone with severe osteoporosis. In later stages of the disease, you can notice kyphosis or a stooped posture. A dowager's hump may develop and there can be neck or back pain due to fractures or bone tenderness. Loss of height can occur - even up to five or six inches.

Reduced bone density can be seen on a DEXA scan, which tests bone mineral density to provide a 'T-score'. The T-score compares bone density to that of a 25-year-old and focuses on the lower spine and hip. A score of -1 to -2.5 indicates osteopenia, which indicates the beginning of osteoporosis. A T-score of more than -2.5 is considered osteoporosis.

Who is at risk?

Bone loss occurs in everyone as we get older. Osteoporosis occurs primarily in older people and in women who have gone through menopause. The leading causes of osteoporosis are decreased estrogen in women at menopause, and lowered testosterone levels in men. If you do not get enough calcium and phosphate, or if your body does not absorb enough calcium, that will hurt bone production and increase your risk.

Some risk factors are controllable and some are not. Women are at higher risk than men. They have smaller bones and may have issues that increase risk such as: late menarche, amenorrhea, and hysterectomy at a young age. Additionally, osteoporosis seems to run in families.

Other risk factors include:

♦   Sustaining a fracture after age 50

♦   Being Caucasian or Asian

♦   Smoking

♦   Being thin

♦   Doing little exercise

♦   A diet without sufficient vitamin D and calcium

♦   Having any of these conditions: rheumatoid arthritis, type 1 diabetes, anorexia, premature menopause, asthma, multiple sclerosis, lupus, and thyroid, gastrointestinal, and blood and renal disorders

♦   Some antacids and cancer treatments

Why is the occurrence of osteoporosis increasing?

Some of the increase in the occurrence of osteoporosis can be attributed to an increase in testing of women over age 50. Lack of physical activity and poor diet is increasing the prevalence of osteoporosis. Only a small percentage of us have jobs that involve physical activity and most people have sedentary lifestyles. Osteoporosis is increasing for many of the same reasons obesity is increasing.

There are medications that help control this disease, but they may have side effects. If you perform weight bearing and resistance exercises and follow a bone healthy diet, you can reduce your chances of developing osteoporosis.

Exercise for Osteoporosis

Exercise is an important component in the treatment of osteoporosis. A well-designed program may help decrease bone loss and the risk of fractures. It is important to focus on exercise that is designed to treat osteoporosis by strengthening bones and muscles leading to better posture and balance. If you have osteoporosis or osteopenia you should understand how to exercise properly and safely to decrease the risk of the progression of the disease. According to the National Osteoporosis Foundation, half of all women and 1 out of 4 men over age 50 will have a wrist, hip, or spine fracture due to osteoporosis. Effective and safe exercise can improve your quality of life, overall health, and keep osteoporosis under control.

How can exercise reduce the risk of osteoporosis?

We lose muscle mass as we age. Less muscle mass leads to less tugging on the bones, and the bones lose density with decreased usage. Not only does strength training increase our muscle mass, which has numerous benefits, it also stimulates the bones and can slow the loss of bone density.

It is a good idea to start building bone mass at a young age. This way you will start with a higher level of bone mass as you age. The activity of bone forming cells begins to decrease at age 35. Weight bearing and resistance exercises are the best exercises for increasing bone density. These types of exercises not only strengthen bones, but also keep your heart healthy, muscles strong, and help with weight control.

What exercises are best for increasing bone density?

An effective exercise program includes weight bearing aerobic exercises, strength training, posture and balance exercise. Weight bearing exercise means the weight of the body is transmitted through the bones. Walking, dancing and hiking are examples of weight bearing exercise. These should be done about five times per week for 45 minutes per session. If you are using a treadmill, hold on to the handles. A recumbent bicycle is ideal because its use eliminates the risk of falling. Do not do high impact exercise, which can cause a fracture. Swimming and water exercises, although good for the heart, are not as effective for increasing bone density.

It's important to focus on exercises designed to treat osteoporosis by strengthening bones and muscles leading to better posture and balance. Strength training or resistance exercise generates muscle tension on the bone.

Strength training actually stimulates the bone because the muscle is pulling on the bone.

To begin strength training, start with a light weight, performing one set of 10 reps. Add weight slowly. Strength training should be done two to three times per week without working the same muscle group two days in a row. Improving muscle strength will also help improve balance. Exercising while standing is more effective and can help with balance as well.

It is important to work on balance training to prevent falls. Falling or the fear of falling is a serious problem for someone with osteoporosis. A fear of falling can cause you to become inactive, which will accelerate your loss of bone mass. Always wear the proper footwear when you exercise. Balance exercises should be performed daily and simply practicing standing on one leg for 10 seconds will help and can be done anywhere. It is important to keep the major muscle groups of the legs and core strong, which will also help improve balance. Recommended balance exercises are listed in Chapter 6.

Postural exercise is also important. A goal is to decrease the risk of rounded shoulders and spinal fractures. Emphasize body awareness and alignment during exercise and activities of daily living. Posture exercises, such as those listed in Chapter 5, can help maintain proper body alignment and can be performed a few times per day. You should be mindful of your posture throughout the day. A good stretching program will help. Focus on stretching the chest muscle and strengthening the back muscles to prevent rounded shoulders. Keeping muscles strong and flexible will also help with spinal stability.

What exercises can potentially cause fractures?

There are precautions to take for osteoporosis. Always keep in mind that bending forward from the waist, side bending and rotation are contraindicated. Doing something as simple as reaching for the toes can be harmful. If you have to bend forward, keep your back straight, and hinge from your hips without rounding your back.

You need to learn how to move in ways that will avoid compression fractures if you have osteoporosis. Try to avoid extreme twisting of the trunk and movements that involve bending forward or rounding your spine; these have been found to increase spinal fractures. Since an abdominal crunch, other traditional abdominal exercises and some abdominal machines are contraindicated, it is necessary to perform other abdominal exercises that do not involve forward flexion. Also, carefully examine the motions involved in sports that you participate in. For example, a golf swing might create too much force for the spine and might have to be modified.

How can you strengthen your core?

It's important to know which exercises are safe to strengthen the core if your bone mass is low. Some examples of exercises that are safe are the pelvic tilt (page 119) and the modified dead bug (page 127).

A large percentage of Pilates and Yoga exercises have to be modified to avoid bending, twisting, and forward bending with rotation. For example, you can do the hundred, double leg stretch, and the crisscross with your head on the floor. There are still many Pilates exercise that can be done without modification, such as single leg circles and the corkscrew (page 128). Spinal extension exercises such as swimming and Pilates back extension exercises may be performed. The posterior of the vertebrae contain cortical bone, which is strong. Therefore, back extension is safe.

Osteoporosis is typically less prevalent in people who are active, and exercise may also prevent osteopenia from becoming osteoporosis. After medical clearance, you can begin to exercise. Warm up before starting, and cool down afterward. You should use proper body mechanics during your exercise sessions and throughout the day. The body needs to always be aligned properly so there is less stress on the spine. This will help you to maintain good posture, which can help improve kyphosis. Try to participate in strength training, posture and balance exercises, and be mindful of your condition during daily activities.

Chapter 9

Lymphedema

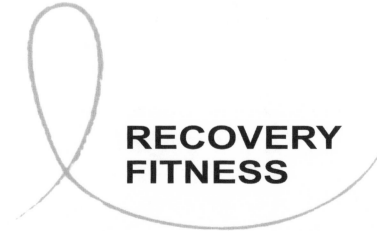

RECOVERY FITNESS

Lymphedema

Lymphedema is a swelling produced by an accumulation of lymph fluid in tissue. Too much lymph fluid can accumulate in an area of the body that has been damaged because of the removal of lymph nodes or radiation to the area. Fibrosis of the axilla due to surgery or radiation can also cause lymphatic obstruction. Symptoms include a feeling of tightness, leathery skin texture, and heaviness. Lymphedema can be debilitating, painful and can affect emotional health.

The circulatory system is made up of arteries, veins and the lymphatic system. The lymphatic system relies on the movement of muscles to circulate the lymph fluid throughout the body. You can think of the lymphatic system as a road system. When one or more roads are blocked due to lymph node removal, the system does not flow smoothly. The "traffic congestion" can cause swelling known as lymphedema.

Even if you have only had a few lymph nodes removed, you should still understand the lymphedema precautions. Lymphedema can occur right after surgery, or years later.

Decreasing the Risk of Lymphedema

One of the most important things you can do to decrease your risk of lymphedema is to keep your weight at a good level. It is also important to learn proper nutrition and the appropriate exercise routines for your specific needs.

The following are additional steps one should take to decrease the chance of developing lymphedema:

♦ Try to avoid extreme temperatures, and avoid sunburns.

♦ Avoid restricting your lymph circulation. Examples of this would be taking blood samples from or blood pressure on the affected arm, carrying a heavy bag on your arm, or wearing tight clothing and jewelry.

♦ Check regularly for infection and call your doctor immediately if an infection occurs. Insect bites, scratches, skin punctures, and bites can cause infections.

♦ Wash the affected area frequently and apply moisturizer to avoid cracks in the skin.

The National Lymphedema Network's website (www.lymphnet.org) is a terrific resource. You should also speak with your therapist for a complete list of lymphedema precautions.

Lymphedema Therapist

Learn the first signs of lymphedema, because it is easier to manage if treated early. Your lymphedema specialist will teach you Complex Decongestive Therapy consisting of skin care, manual lymph drainage and exercise. If you meet with your lymphedema specialist at the first signs of swelling, pitting, redness, heaviness, etc., lymphedema can be kept under control. The specialist will also make sure that your exercise plan is compatible with the treatment and will clear you to exercise if your lymphedema is under control.

Additionally, if baseline measurements have not already been taken at the hospital, it is recommended that you obtain a baseline girth measurement by a lymphedema specialist. The limbs that are at risk for lymphedema should be periodically measured to make sure they have not changed in size. Symptoms can be managed more easily if dealt with as soon as they appear.

A compression garment or sleeve, which supports the muscles and helps bring the lymphatic fluid to the heart, can be worn while exercising and at other times. These garments need to be professionally fitted and monitored by a lymphedema specialist.

Exercise and Lymphedema

Your body will work better if you are engaged in regular physical activity. Moreover, exercise is very helpful for lymphedema control, but it must be done in a safe manner if lymph nodes have been removed or radiated. If you have lymphedema, you should begin to exercise under professional guidance after receiving medical clearance. It is important to learn the right exercises for your particular situation, and how to perform them properly and with good form. Exercise needs to progress slowly using a properly fitted garment. Our goal is to promote physical activity without incurring pain or injury, which can make lymphedema worse.

All of the exercises in this book incorporate abdominal breathing and relaxation breathing. These breathing techniques are beneficial because they:

♦ Stimulate lymph flow and lymphatic drainage

♦ Act as a lymphatic system pump, moving the sluggish lymph fluid

- Enable oxygen to get to the tissues

- Reduce stress, a common cancer side effect

It is also helpful to incorporate Pilates into your exercise routine because of the deep breathing used with each movement. When you begin Pilates exercises, perform just a few repetitions and use no weight, or the lightest machine tension. After you are able to exercise for several sessions without flare-ups, you can use resistance bands, light weights, and modified body weight exercises.

You can develop a good fitness level without triggering lymphedema. Swimming is a very good exercise for those with lymphedema. The water creates compression. Since repetitive motions are risky, try to vary your swimming strokes. The water should not be hot and the pool area should be clean to help you to avoid infection. When you leave the water, follow proper skin care precautions. Moisturize to prevent dry skin which can lead to cracks in the skin and infection.

Yoga poses can cause flare-ups. Do not perform the following poses: downward facing dog, upward facing dog, plank, and side plank. Avoid hot yoga.

Exercise helps the lymphatic fluid to move throughout the body. Muscles pump and push the lymph fluid and can help move the lymph away from the affected area. Strength training may help pump the lymph fluid away from the affected limb, but it does not necessarily prevent lymphedema. Slow progression of exercise will allow you to monitor fullness or aching, which can indicate stress to the lymphatic system. You should stop if you feel tired or if your limb aches or feels heavy. Please read the strength training information in Chapter 4 prior to beginning a strength training routine.

Chapter 10

Fitness After Breast, Gynecological and Prostate Cancer

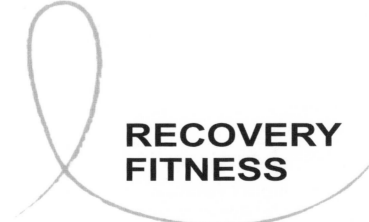

RECOVERY
FITNESS

Fitness after Breast Cancer

I recommend that prior to surgery you have a full fitness assessment. This way, after surgery you have a basis for comparison. Posture is an important component of the evaluation. Often posture is affected by surgery. As a consequence, protective posturing occurs, which is when you limit your range of motion to dodge discomfort.

After a mastectomy, upper cross syndrome or cervical crossed syndrome is a common side effect. A survivor with these symptoms exhibits rounded shoulders, a hunched over upper back, and a head forward position. This develops because some of the muscles become tight and shortened and some become weak and lengthened.

Pain after a surgical procedure is also common, especially in the area where the surgery was performed. Moreover, the recovery process can be complicated because your nerves may have been cut, or you may experience tightening caused by scarring and adhesions.

Surgical Procedures and Appropriate Exercises

The following is a list of the common surgical options, potential side effects in relation to exercise, and the exercises that are helpful when recovering from each surgery. Exercises and activities that are considered unsafe will also be discussed.

Axillary Lymph Node Dissection

Axillary lymph node dissection and radiation increase your risk of lymphedema (see Chapter 9 for detailed information on lymphedema). Lymphedema can happen directly after surgery or many years later. Contact your doctor if you notice swelling, or fullness or heaviness in the arm or any body part. Other warning signs are tight jewelry and clothing, and redness or warmth in the area of concern.

Axillary lymph node dissection also may cause you to develop cording or axillary web syndrome, which looks like a vertical cord under the skin. Cording forms when tendons or lymphatic channels stick to the underside of skin where there is scar tissue from the lymph node dissection. See a lymphedema specialist or physical therapist if this occurs.

A lymphedema therapist or physician needs to be seen if you have lymphedema. Decongestive and breathing exercises are an important part of lymphedema management. Once you have your lymphedema under control and receive medical clearance, you can proceed with the gentle exercises in this book.

The serratus muscle can also be affected by surgery, which presents as winging or protraction of the scapula. You must strengthen the serratus anterior and increase its ability to stabilize the scapula.

Important exercises are the Serratus Reach (page 77) and the Wall Push-Up with scapular protraction (page 130). Your goal is to regain range of motion and then strengthen by following the exercises in this book.

Lumpectomy & Mastectomy without Reconstruction

The discomfort from the pain and tightness in the area of the incision can cause poor posture. As a result, rather than try to correct poor posture, sufferers will adopt a form of protective, but incorrect posture such as a head forward position (not in line with the body) and shoulders that are hunched or rounded forward. Radiation can shorten and stiffen the pectoral muscles.

Your exercise plan should involve prevention of upper cross syndrome, which is a muscle imbalance that can lead to head, neck and back pain. It alters your posture and creates a whole set of additional problems. If this syndrome applies to you it will be necessary for you to follow the exercises that stretch the tight muscles and strengthen the weak muscles. These include stretches that loosen the pectorals and neck area and exercises that strengthen the rhomboids and lower traps. Your goal is to regain your range of motion and then strengthen your muscles by following the exercises in this book.

Reconstructive Surgery

Implant Surgery

During implant reconstruction, and during tissue expansions, the pectoralis major is pushed away from the ribs. This can affect range of motion and posture. Protective posturing occurs, which is when you limit your range of motion to dodge discomfort.

Potential side effects from implant reconstruction

Inactivity and protective posturing can lead to a frozen shoulder, which may become permanent unless you start to stretch.

You need to stretch the tight muscles: upper trapezius, scapula, pectorals.

You need to strengthen the weak muscles: anterior neck flexors, rhomboids, lower trapezius, serratus.

Axillary lymph node dissection and radiation can cause weakness and tightness of different muscle groups. In addition to causing a head forward, rounded shoulders posture, your range of motion of the shoulder can be affected. These symptoms may be worsened by reconstructive surgeries. It will be important for you to do all the stretches in the book that stretch the shoulder: flexion, extension and abduction. It is also important to stretch and strengthen the muscles of the rotator cuff.

Avoid: Military push-ups and chest press with very heavy weights (not advised without additional medical clearance).

TRAM Flap Surgery

A TRAM (transverse rectus abdominis myocutaneous) flap consists of skin, fat, rectus muscle, and blood vessels taken from the abdominal wall and transferred to the chest to reconstruct the breast. Initially, it was a pedicled flap, then with the advent of microsurgery, it became a free flap. The fat, blood and rectus abdominus are pulled through a tunnel that is created under the skin to form a breast mound or a pocket for a breast implant. This may disturb surrounding tissue. The abdominal muscles are rotated to the chest.

The rectus abdominus supports and stabilizes the spine. Weakness in this area can pave the way for back problems. Your rectus muscle helps you maintain good posture and bend forward. This core muscle plays a role in strength, posture, balance and flexibility. TRAM flap surgery can weaken the foundation or core of the body and is being replaced by newer techniques.

Potential side effects from TRAM flap surgery

1. Posture: With the diminished support from the abdominal wall, it may be difficult to stand erect and you may develop *lordosis*, an inward curvature of the spine. You may also suffer from abdominal and lower back weakness.

   Our goal is for you to regain range of motion and then strengthen by following the exercises in this book.

2. Flexibility: Upper and lower body flexibility may be compromised. You

may find tightness in the hip flexors. This is due to leaning forward as a result of tightness from abdominal surgery.

All of the stretches in this book should be performed. Make sure you include the hip flexor stretch (page 101).

3. Balance: Your balance may be affected due to a decrease in core

   strength. Perform balance exercises such as front, side, and back leg lifts (pages 131-132) and engage in core strengthening.

4. Core Strength: Exercise must be done to improve core strength. The rectus abdominus stabilizes the spine. Since it is no longer in the same place, other muscles have to work harder to compensate for the change. It is crucial to focus on strengthening the obliques and back muscles. Because the back can be vulnerable to injury, it is necessary to learn how to lift properly.

   Exercises to strengthen the core: Pelvic Tilt (page 119), and modified Pilates exercises (page 128). Exhaling while pressing the belly button to the spine will help to strengthen the transverse abdominals. During core strengthening on the floor, use the band to control the intensity of the exercise.

   Exercises to strengthen the obliques: Cross-Over Crunch (page 125), Lateral Crunch (page 125), Side Knee Drops (page 126).

   Exercises to strengthen the back: Bridge (page 120), Bird Dog (page 123), and the other back strengthening exercises demonstrated in this book.

   There are some exercises that are contraindicated such as sit-ups or any forceful movement to the abdominal area. In addition, heavy lifting should be avoided to minimize the risk of a hernia.

DIEP Flap Surgery

A DIEP flap is a refined version of a TRAM flap that spares the muscle. The blood vessels are dissected from the rectus abdominis muscle.

The advantage to DIEP flap breast reconstruction is that the rectus abdominis muscle is not moved, so the risk of abdominal weakness or hernia is decreased. This surgical technique decreases negative side effects of the TRAM flap such as back trouble and issues with posture and balance.

The goal is to regain range of motion and then strengthen by following the exercises in this book.

Latissimus Dorsi Flap Surgery

In this reconstructive surgery, latissimus dorsi muscle tissue in the upper back is rotated to the chest, possibly disturbing surrounding tissue. The latissimus dorsi muscle allows the shoulder to rotate, helps to keep the scapula flat, and adducts the arm.

Potential side effects from latissimus dorsi flap surgery

The shoulder and back may become weaker and some women have difficulties with maintaining proper posture . Posture must be corrected first before strengthening the area. Good posture and flexibility take precedence over strength training, to ensure proper biomechanics and form. You must stretch the chest muscles and strengthen the back and shoulder muscles.

The goal is to regain range of motion and then strengthen by following the exercises in this book.

Exercises that will help lat flap surgery:

♦ Serratus Reach (page 77)

♦ Chest Flies: Lie flat on your back with your knees bent and your feet flat on the floor. Hold a dumbbell in each hand if you are using weight (no weight to start). Open your arms to the side with your palms facing the ceiling. This is your starting position. Inhale to start, then exhale as you raise your arms up so that they are directly over your chest, palms/ weights facing one another. Perform 5-10 reps.

♦ Reverse Fly (page 135)

♦ Upper back strengthening using the band: Rows (page 139) and Lat Pull-Downs (page 140), with an emphasis on the rhomboids and trapezius.

♦ Rotator Cuff Exercises (page 140)

Avoid: pull-ups and lat pull-downs with very heavy weight.

Fitness after Gynecological Cancer

Exercise will help increase blood flow to the affected area, accelerating the healing process. As soon as possible after surgery, start walking and deep breathing. Place your hands on your abdomen, inhale and fill your torso with air, then slowly exhale through the mouth while contracting the abdominal muscles. This can be done while sitting, standing, or lying in bed.

Flexibility of the pelvis, torso, and hips can be compromised after gynecological cancer surgery and treatments. Try to perform flexibility stretches 1-3 times per day. Hold each stretch for 5-10 seconds and gradually work up to performing 5-10 reps.

Initial Helpful Stretches

Exercise	Page
The Arch and Curl: In supine position, press the shoulders into the floor and arch the middle back off the floor. Hold for 3 seconds, then press the abdominals to the floor, allowing the shoulders to come off the floor.	n/a
Cobra: Lie prone propped up on your forearms.	n/a
Pelvic Tilt	119
Bridge	120

Additional Standing Stretches

Exercise	Page
Standing Cat Stretch	85
Alternating Reach	86
Rope Climbing	86
Side Stretch	87
Tai Chi Inspired Stretch	97
Side and IT Band Stretch	98
Waitress Stretch	100
Overhead Stretch	101

Additional Floor Stretches

Exercise	Page
Stretching Rack	105
Knee Drop	106
Spinal Rotation (Shoulder Opener and Torso Stretch)	107
Child's Pose	109
Cat/Cow	109
Seated Butterfly	110
Seated Hip Stretch	110
Shoulder and Torso Stretch	112
Stretches on the Large Exercise Ball	115-116

Whenever muscles are cut it results in weakness. The following exercises will help you to restore strength. Improve slowly and review the strength training precautions in Chapter 1.

Strength Building Exercises

Exercise	Page
Pelvic Tilt	119
Bridge	120
Superman	122
Alternating Superman	122
Bird Dog and Variations	123-124
Abdominal Exercises	119-128
Wall Sit and Wall Sit with the Large Exercise Ball	129 & 141
Plié Wall Sit with the Large Exercise Ball	142

Fitness after Prostate Cancer

The muscle that surrounds the prostate may be weakened from cancer surgery and treatments. You may become incontinent, with less control over your urine flow.

Kegel exercises strengthen your pelvic floor muscles to control urine flow. The pelvic floor muscles are comprised of the bladder, sphincter and the pubococcyges muscle. These muscles are used to stop the flow of urine.

Women are often advised to practice Kegels before and after childbirth, but Kegels are also great for prostate cancer patients because they minimize incontinence and can improve erectile issues. They can help control incontinence without medication or surgery. It is wise to start Kegel exercises before surgery and treatments.

You can find your pelvic floor muscles by squeezing your sphincter and contracting the urethra to stop the flow of urine when using the bathroom.

Kegel Exercise

Perform the Kegel 10 times holding for 5 seconds each. Try to do this four times per day. Take a 5-second break between each repetition. It may take several weeks or months to be able to contract your muscles for 5 seconds at a time, or to repeat it 10 times. If you perform the Kegel several times per day, your pelvic floor strength should improve.

Tips

- Try not to use the surrounding muscle groups in the buttocks, legs and abdomen.
- Try to lift the pelvic floor upward.
- You can perform this exercise in any position: standing, sitting, or lying in bed.
- Kegels can be done at any time, such as while watching TV, waiting in line or driving.

Chapter 11

Upper Body Stretching

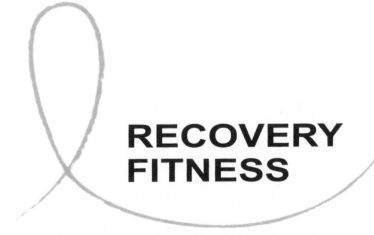

RECOVERY FITNESS

Upper Body Stretching

The exercises in this chapter focus on relaxing and lengthening the muscles in your upper body to help you achieve greater comfort and a wider range of motion. These stretches may be performed either standing or sitting and each should be done with relaxation breathing. To practice relaxation breathing, slowly inhale through the nose for 5 seconds, and then slowly exhale through the mouth for 5 seconds.

Neck Stretches

Neck Rotation

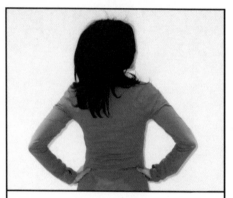

Slowly inhale and turn your head over the right shoulder. Hold and slowly exhale, then return your head back to center. Do the same on the left side.

Lateral Neck Stretch

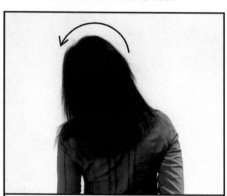

Slowly inhale and tilt your left ear down toward the left shoulder. Hold and slowly exhale, then return your head to center. Do the same on the right side.

Neck Stretch Variation

Place your hands behind your back with the fingers interlaced. Bring your hands to the right hip and bring the elbows together and the right ear to the right shoulder. Hold for 5 seconds, then do the same on the left side.

"Double Chin" Neck Stretch

Look down toward your chest and pull your head and neck slightly back. Hold the stretch through a cycle of relaxation breathing. This stretch helps to counteract the postural habit many of us do unconsciously: a head forward posture.

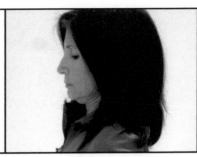

Shoulder Stretches

Shoulder Shrug

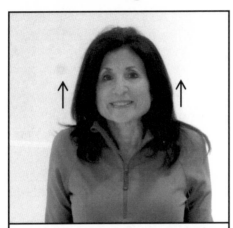

Raise your shoulders up toward your ears, while inhaling slowly for 5 seconds. Press your shoulders all the way back down, while exhaling slowly for 5 seconds.

Tip: Perform all exercises with good posture. If standing, your feet should be hip-width apart and your knees should not be locked.

Backward Shoulder Roll

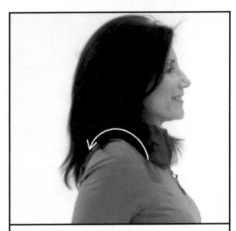

Raise your shoulders up toward your ears, while inhaling slowly for 5 seconds. Slowly roll your shoulders backward and press them all the way back down, while exhaling slowly for 5 seconds. Increase the size of the circle with each roll.

Variation: Reverse the direction to roll your shoulders forward.

Scapular Retraction

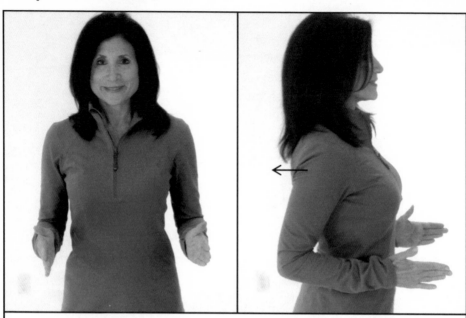

Hold your arms at your sides, elbows bent to create a 90° angle. Firmly squeeze your shoulder blades together as you draw your shoulders and elbows back. Focus on squeezing your shoulder blades together as if trying to hold a walnut between them, then release to the starting position.

Serratus Reach

Hold your arms out in front of you, parallel to the floor, palms facing the floor. Gently pull your shoulders forward. Try to focus on initiating the movement from your shoulders rather than reaching with your fingertips. Let your fingertips move forward as a result of reaching with the shoulders.

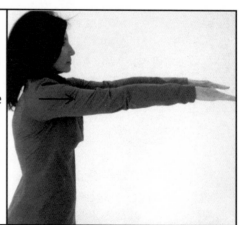

Posterior Shoulder Stretch with Neck Rotation

Bring your right arm across your body, using your left arm to pull it toward your chest (pictured). Hold your arm back above or below the elbow, rather than putting direct pressure on the elbow joint. Slowly turn your head over the right shoulder. Slowly inhale for 5 seconds, then slowly exhale for 5 seconds, returning your head and arms to the neutral starting position. Repeat the stretch and rotation on the left side.

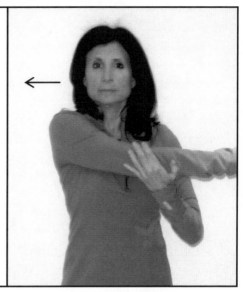

Shoulder Abduction

Starting with arms straight down at your sides, palms facing the body, slowly raise one arm to the side, palm facing the floor. Try to raise the arm 180°, but never to the point of pain. Slowly lower the arm back to your side. Repeat with your opposite arm. Repeat with both arms simultaneously. Try to slightly increase the height to which you can raise your arm each time you perform this stretch. You should feel tension in the stretch, but stop if you begin to feel pain.

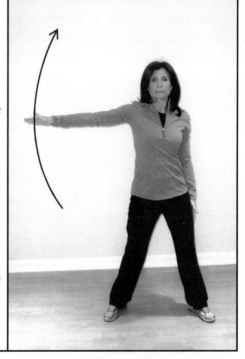

Shoulder Flexion

Starting with your arms straight down at your sides, slowly raise one arm in front of the body, palm facing the floor. Try to raise the arm 180°, but never to the point of pain. Slowly lower the arm back to your side. Repeat with the opposite arm. Repeat on each side, increasing your range of motion with each stretch. You may not be able to raise the arm 180° at first, but slowly build your range of motion as you stretch on a regular basis. You should feel tension, but not pain.

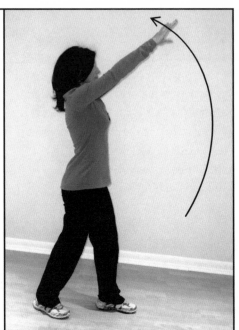

Shoulder Flexion with Additional Held Stretch

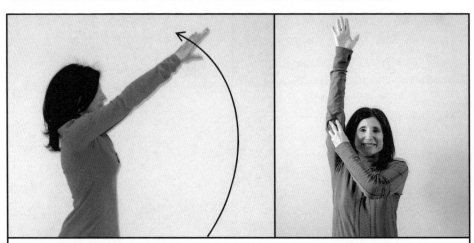

Perform the shoulder flexion stretch above, and when the working arm is raised to its highest position, gently push back on that arm with the opposite hand just until you feel some tension. Hold the stretch while performing two cycles of relaxation breathing.

Shoulder Flexion with Fist Pump

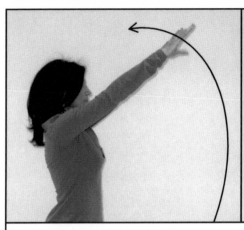 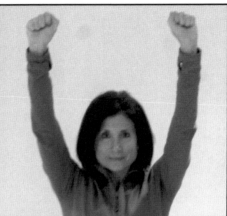

Perform the shoulder flexion stretch with both arms simultaneously, and when your arms are raised to their highest position, gently squeeze your hands to make fists. Release the fists and lower your arms back to your sides. Performing the fist pump encourages the flow of lymphatic fluid.

Shoulder Flexion Against the Wall

This is a classic "Finger Walking" exercise: Turn to face the wall, standing about a foot away from the wall. You may need to stand a bit farther away from the wall at first. Please your arm at your side with your elbow bent to about 90° and with your fingers gently touching the wall. Slowly walk your fingers up the wall, as high as you can comfortably go, with the goal of fully extending your arm overhead. Slowly walk your fingers back down the wall again to the starting position. Repeat on the opposite side. This is one of the first exercises recommended after breast surgery and lymph node dissection.

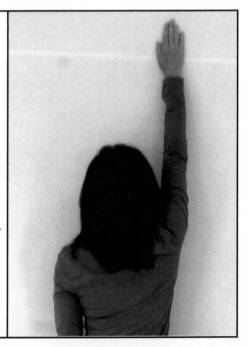

Shoulder Extension with Chest Lift Variations

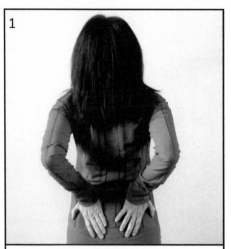

1

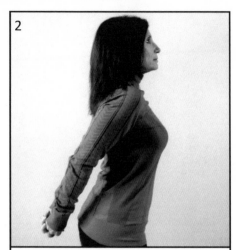

2

Bring both arms behind your back with elbows bent, placing your hands in the small of your back. Hold for a cycle of relaxation breathing. This stretch combines shoulder extension, adduction and medial rotation.

Lower your arms to your sides. Reach your arms behind your back and clasp your hands together, gently pulling your arms away from your body. Hold for a cycle of relaxation breathing. This will also stretch your chest.

Shoulder Extension with Forward Lean

Stand with your legs hip-width apart and clasp your hands together behind your back. Slowly hinge forward, ending in a table-top flat back position. Gently lift your arms up behind your back, keeping your hands clasped. Try to keep your neck and head in line with your spine in a neutral position, rather than letting them drop toward the floor. Hold the stretch for a cycle of relaxation breathing, then release and return to an upright position.

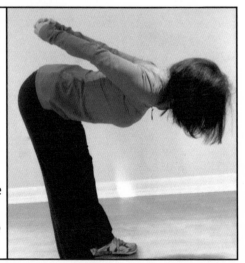

Pendulum Stretch

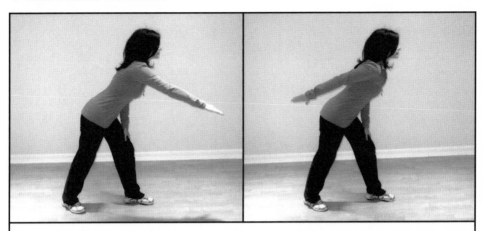

Stand with one leg in front of the other, torso slightly hinged forward, allowing one arm to hang down. Slowly swing the arm forward and back, increasing the range of motion slightly with each swing. Repeat the stretch on the opposite side.

Variation: Swing both arms together, forward and back. Variation 2: Rest one arm on a table and let the other arm hang down. Slowly swing the arm front to back, side to side and then in circles.

Cross-Body Swing

Stand with your legs together, knees slightly bent, and torso slightly hinged forward. Let one arm hang down. Slowly swing the working arm across your body and then away from your body, increasing the range of motion slightly with each swing. Repeat the stretch on the opposite side.

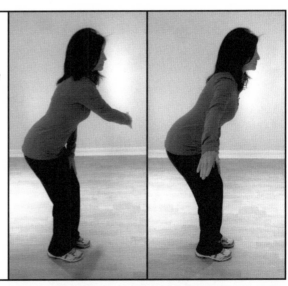

The Scapular Clock

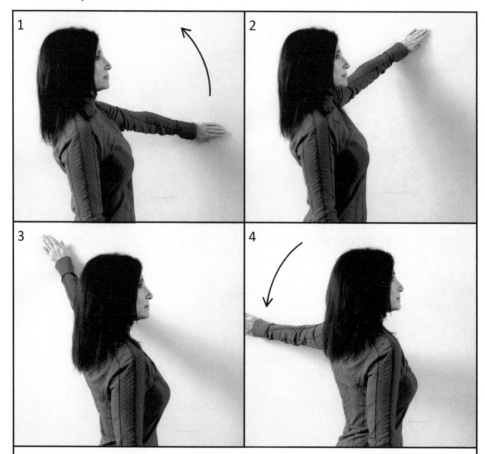

Stand with your side to the wall and the palm of your hand closest to the wall pressed flat against it. Point your fingers to the 3 o'clock position (image 1). Press firmly against the wall for 10 seconds, then slowly walk your fingers up the wall counterclockwise to the to the 2 o'clock position. Again press your palm firmly against the wall for 10 seconds. Repeat this motion for each hour on the clock, finishing at the 9 o'clock position (image 4). Keep the scapula (shoulder blades) retracted throughout the exercise.

Horizontal Adduction Clock

Facing the wall, bring one arm across the front of your body with the palm of your hand on the wall. The arm should vary in positions 9, 11, 12 o'clock.

Chest Stretches

Pectoral Wall Stretch

Stand with your side to the wall with your right shoulder a few inches away from the wall. Place your right palm on the wall slightly above shoulder height with your elbow bent. Pressing your palm firmly against the wall, gently turn your body away from the wall until you feel a stretch across your chest. Hold the stretch through a cycle of relaxation breathing, then release and repeat on the opposite side.

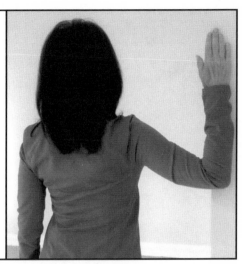

Twisting Pectoral Stretch

Stand with your side to the wall. Place your right palm on the wall at shoulder height with your elbow only slightly bent. Pressing your palm firmly against the wall, and keeping your arm almost straight, gently turn your torso away from the wall until you feel a stretch across your chest. Hold the stretch through a cycle of relaxation breathing, then release and repeat on the opposite side.

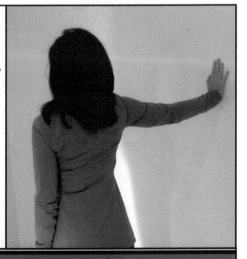

Tracking Your Progress: After the Twisting Pectoral Stretch, remain standing perpendicular to the wall and walk your fingers up the wall. Mark your arm height. Try to go a bit farther each time you perform the stretch.

"VW" Stretch

Stand with your back to the wall and your elbows bent to form a "W" with palms facing forward. While keeping your shoulders and arms flat against the wall, slowly slide your arms up the wall until they form a "V". Inhale for 5 seconds as you slide your arms up the wall, and exhale for 5 seconds as you slide them back down to the "W" position.

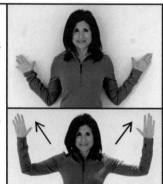

Standing Cat Stretch

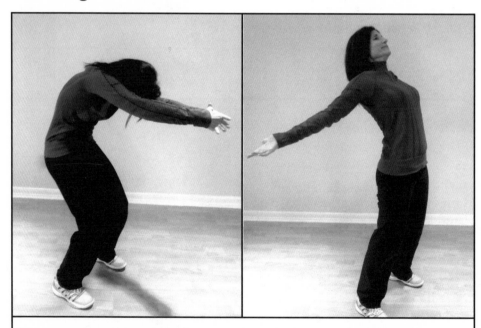

Standing with feet a little wider than shoulder width apart, bring your arms forward, bend your knees and arch your back, pulling your naval toward your spine and tucking your chin to your chest. Slowly unfold from this position and reverse the arch in your back, gently lifting your chest and chin toward the ceiling and extending your arms out behind you.

Additional Upper Body Stretches

Alternating Reach

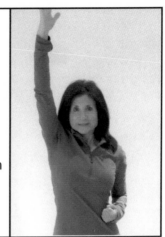

Reach up as high overhead as you can with one arm, while holding the opposite arm at your waist, hand closed in a fist. Reverse to reach up with the opposite arm. Repeat the alternating reach, trying to stretch a little bit farther with every reach.

Variation: Perform the stretch reaching up as high overhead as you can with one arm, while the opposite arm reaches toward the floor.

Climbing the Wall

Face the wall and walk your fingers up as high as possible. It is motivating to mark your finger height on the wall and watch it increase weekly. You can also do this turned so that your affected side is facing the wall.

Rope Climb

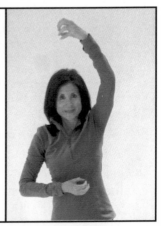

Imagine that you are holding on to a rope that is hanging from the ceiling in front of you. "Grip" the rope with one hand overhead and one hand in front of your waist. Reach as high as possible with the top hand, allowing your torso to lean slightly to the side as you stretch up to "grab" the rope as high as possible. Reverse to "grab" the rope with the opposite hand. Continue "climbing," trying to reach a little higher with each stretch.

Arm Circles

Inhale as you reach both arms high overhead, crossing your wrists at the top. Exhale as you slowly press your arms back, around and down, creating large half circles as your arms come down to your sides. Repeat the stretch, trying to make your circles as large as possible and increasing your range of motion with each circle you make to open your chest and shoulders.

Variation: This stretch may also be performed using one arm at a time in an alternating backstroke motion.

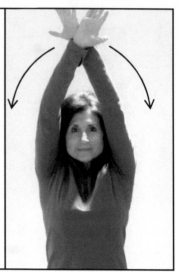

Side Stretch

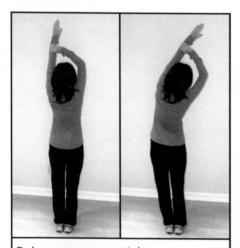

Raise one arm straight up overhead. Hold on to that arm below your wrist with the opposite hand. Tilt gently to the side, maintaining your arm position. Return to center and repeat on the opposite side.

Side Stretch Variations

Variation 1

Perform the side stretch with one arm overhead and the opposite hand behind your lower back.

Variation 2

Perform the side stretch as a lateral bend with your hands behind your ears and your elbows out to the sides. Bend to the side and hold the stretch for 5 seconds, then bend to the other side and hold the stretch for 5 seconds. Afterward, make circles with your elbows, keeping your hands near your ears.

Swimming Stretch: Front Crawl

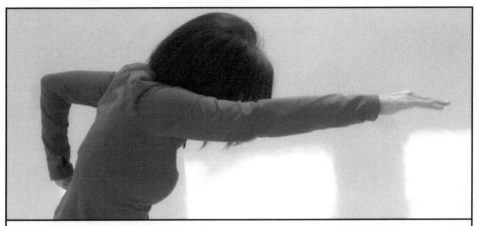

Imagine you are swimming the front crawl. Hinge forward slightly from the hips and reach forward as far as you can with your right arm while pulling your left arm back with a bent elbow. Reverse to reach forward with your left arm while pulling your right arm back with a bent elbow. Move through the stretch fluidly as if pushing through water, and breathe slowly and rhythmically throughout the motions.

Swimming Stretch: Breaststroke

Imagine you are swimming the breaststroke. Hinge forward slightly from the hips and begin with your hands together in front of your chest. Open your hands out to the sides and reach forward with both arms with the elbows slightly bent (shown). Push your arms out to the sides and bring your hands back into your chest to the starting position. Move through the stretch fluidly as if pushing through water, and breathe slowly and rhythmically throughout the motions.

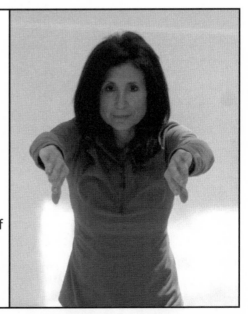

Pectoral and Shoulder Stretch

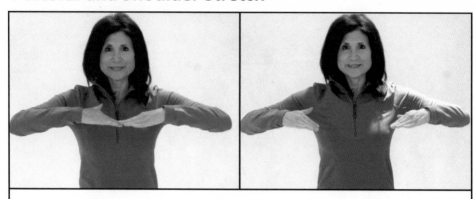

This stretch combines pectoral and shoulder stretching with scapular retraction. Start with your elbows lifted out to the side, parallel to the floor, with your palms facing downward and fingertips just touching. Gently squeeze your shoulder blades backward to open your chest until your hands are in front of your shoulders. Do not let your elbows drop.

Forearm Rotation

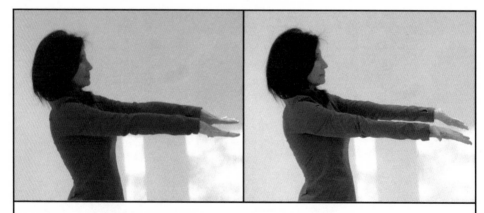

Reach your arms straight out in front of you, parallel to the floor with your palms facing the floor. Slowly rotate your forearms outward until your palms are facing the ceiling. Slowly rotate your forearms inward until your palms are back in the starting position facing the floor.

Variation: Perform the Forearm Rotation with your arms out to the sides. Afterwards, inhale and make fists, then exhale and slowly open the hands.

"Traffic Cop" Rotator Cuff Stretch

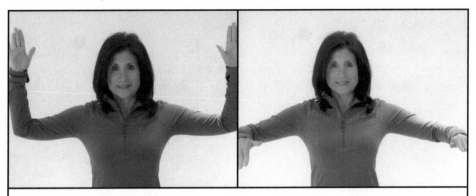

Raise your arms with your elbows bent at a 90° angle, palms facing forward. Rotate your arms down toward the floor until your palms are facing down and your forearms are parallel to the floor.

Bent Elbow Arm Raise

Clasp your hands together at chest level with bent elbows out to the side, keeping your shoulders down and back. Raise your arms up to head level.

Lymphatic Fluid Stimulation Stretch

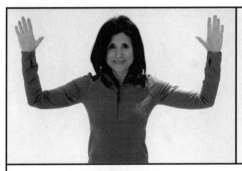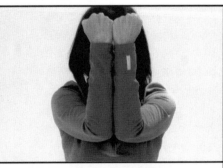

Raise your arms with your elbows bent at a 90° angle, palms facing forward. Maintaining their height, rotate your arms inward until your elbows meet in front of your chest. Squeeze your hands in to fists. Making fists is important as this helps stimulate the flow of lymphatic fluid.

Variation: This can also be done in prayer position, palm to palm at chest level. Inhale, then exhale as you press the palms together for 5 seconds.

Triceps Stretch

Raise one arm and touch the back of your shoulder with your hand. Gently lift and press the arm up with the opposite hand. Hold the stretch for a cycle of relaxation breathing, then release and repeat on the opposite side. The higher you lift your arm, the deeper stretch you will feel in your triceps.

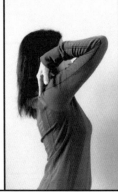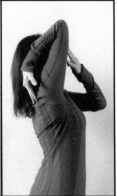

Archery Stretch

Reach both arms forward. Pull one elbow back, initiating the movement from your shoulder blade, while the other arm stays forward. Do the same for the other arm.

Two-Handed Back Scratch

Hold a resistance band or towel between your hands, with your hands down at your sides. Be sure that the band/towel crosses behind your back rather than in front of you. Bend your elbows and slowly slide your hands up your back as high as possible (shown), bringing both the shoulders and elbows back. Hold the stretch through a cycle of relaxation breathing, then slowly slide your hands back down to your sides. Do not pull or stretch the band/towel. It is only used to maintain your arm spacing.

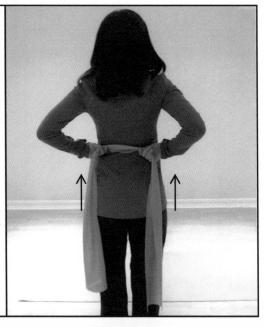

Upper Body Stretches with a Cane

The following stretches use a cane to aid with arm placement and movement. Although the curved handle of a cane serves as a convenient and comfortable grip, you may use a broom, stick or rod in place of the cane.

Shoulder Flexion with Cane

Hold the top of a cane or a stick in one hand with that arm raised straight up, holding the bottom of the cane in the other hand with that arm across your waist. Gently press your top arm back and slightly out to the side, then return to the starting position. Repeat on the opposite side.

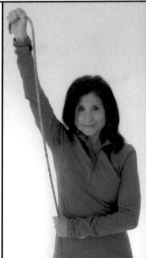
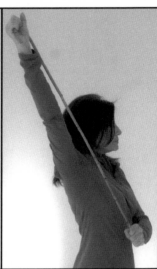

Shoulder Flexion with Cane Variation

Hold the cane in front of your body in both hands with your hands hip-width apart on the cane. Gently raise the cane up as high as you can until a point of tension, but not pain. Hold the stretch through a cycle of relaxation breathing, then slowly lower the cane back down.

Kayak Stretch

Hold a cane or a stick in front of you with both hands. Imagine that you are holding a kayak paddle and row with the cane by dipping one end down to the side, then lifting that side and dipping the other side down. Let each stroke get larger and larger. This stretch can be done sitting or standing.

Shoulder Extension with Cane

Hold a cane or stick behind your back in both hands with your hands hip-width apart on the cane. Gently raise the cane, extending your arms away from your back as high as you can until a point of tension, but not pain (shown). Hold the stretch through a cycle of relaxation breathing, then slowly lower the cane back to the starting position. Note: this stretch may be done with a band or a towel in place of the cane.

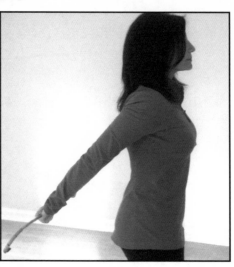

Diagonal Cane Stretch (Chest)

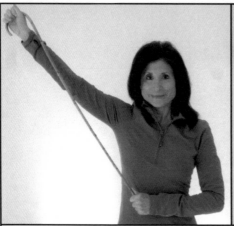
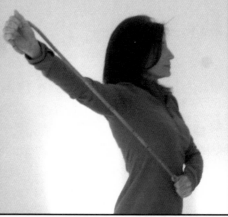

Hold the top of a cane or a stick in one hand with that arm raised up on a diagonal, holding the bottom of the cane in the other hand with that arm across your waist. Gently press the extended arm out on the diagonal to open up your chest. Hold the stretch through a cycle of relaxation breathing, then slowly return to the starting position. Repeat on the opposite side. Note: this stretch may also be performed with the cane reaching out to the side, rather than on a high diagonal.

Back Scratch Stretch with Cane

Hold the cane behind your back with one arm holding the bottom of the cane and the other arm holding the cane closer to the top (shown). Keep both your elbows and your shoulders back. Pull up with the top arm and allow the bottom arm to move up as you pull. Then pull down with the bottom arm and allow the top arm to move down as you pull. Hold at the maximum pain free range at each of the top and bottom stretches for 10 seconds, building up to 30 seconds. Breathe slowly throughout the stretch.

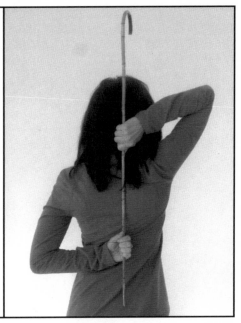

Chapter 12

Total Body Stretching: Standing

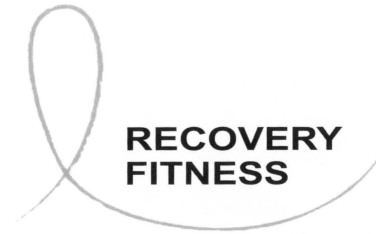

RECOVERY FITNESS

Total Body Stretching: Standing

The stretches in this chapter will engage more than one muscle group at a time, and are designed to be performed in a standing position. Continue to do relaxation breathing as you gently work through each stretch.

Tai Chi Inspired Stretch

Tai Chi combines physical movement with mental concentration. This exercise uses gentle rhythmic movement coordinated with breathing. It works on dynamic or moving balance as you shift your weight from leg to leg while moving the arms.

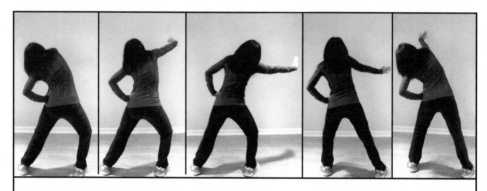

Begin in a wide stance with your weight centered.

Using the right arm, shown:
As you shift your weight on to the right leg and bend the right knee, the right elbow reaches to the right. As you shift to the left leg, the right palm reaches to the left and pushes away from the body.

Using the left arm:
As you shift your weight on to the left leg and bend the left knee, the left elbow reaches to the left . As you shift to the right leg, the left palm reaches to the right and pushes away from the body.

Stretches with Wall Assistance

Side and IT Band Stretch

Stand next to a sturdy column. If a pole or column is not available, you may use a doorknob on a closed door, standing on the outside of the door if it opens in to a room (you do not want to accidentally open the door while using the knob for support). With your side to the column/door, hold on with your inside arm and cross your outside foot over your supporting foot, reaching it toward the column/door. Reach up overhead with your outside arm and slowly lean away from the column/door, holding on for support. Press your hips to the outside, reaching in opposition with your arm and crossed-over foot. You will feel a deep side stretch as well as a stretch in your iliotibial (IT) band. Hold for two cycles of relaxation breathing then do the stretch on the other side.

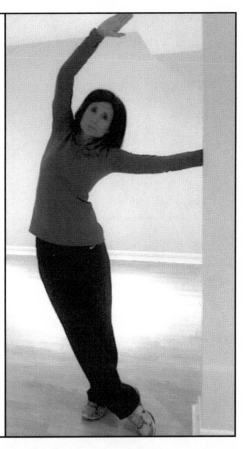

Tip: Imagine a traffic light for pain perception. If during and following a stretch you do not feel any pain, you have a green light to continue performing that stretch during your next training session. If during a stretch you do not feel pain, but afterward pain develops, you have a yellow light to proceed with caution with that stretch, reducing your range of motion during the stretch until pain is no longer felt afterward. If you feel pain during a stretch, you have a red light and should reduce your range of motion immediately.

Calf Stretch

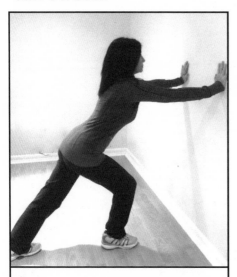

Stand about a foot away from the wall. Press your palms against the wall and step backward with one leg, bending your front knee and keeping your back leg straight. Hold for a cycle of relaxation breathing then reverse.

Quad Stretch

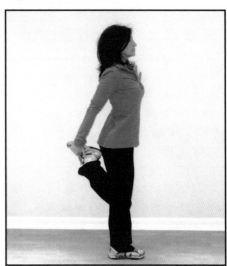

Stand with your side to the wall, placing a hand on the wall for balance. Hold your outside foot with your outside hand and lift the foot up toward your rear end, keeping your thighs and knees together. Hold for a cycle of relaxation breathing then reverse.

Standing Figure 4 Hip Stretch

Stand with your side to the wall, placing a hand on the wall for balance. With one leg slightly bent, rotate the opposite hip so that your other foot can rest on the weight-bearing knee. Gently lower your bottom as if starting to sit back in to a chair, maintaining your crossed leg position. Engage your abdominals for support. Hold for a cycle of relaxation breathing then reverse.

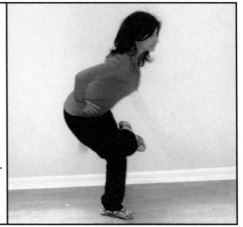

Stretches without Wall Assistance

Waitress Stretch

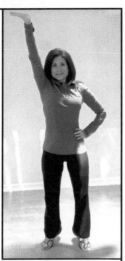

Imagine that you're balancing a platter on top of one hand. Reach the working arm up while rising up on the balls of your feet. Press your palm to the ceiling.

Lengthen your entire body from your wrist to your toes and hold the position for 10-30 seconds. Slowly lower your heels to the floor. Reverse by reaching up with the opposite arm. If you are not able to balance unassisted, you may gently hold on to a chair back or the wall with the resting hand.

Hamstring & Calf Stretch

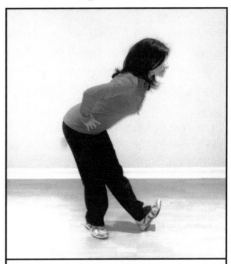

Place one foot in front of you and hinge at the waist to lean your torso forward toward the leg that is extended (shown), and bend your supporting knee. Slowly flex your front ankle so that your toes are pulling up toward your body. Hold for a cycle of relaxation breathing then reverse.

Inner Thigh Stretch

Place one leg out to the side with a flexed foot. Bend your supporting knee and hinge at the waist to lean your torso forward, pressing your hips back. Hold for a cycle of relaxation breathing, then shift your weight to the other side to reverse.

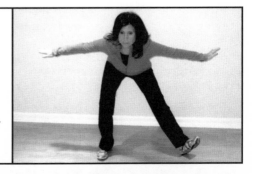

Hip Flexor Stretch

Lunge forward with your right foot, bending your right knee no farther than 90° and lowering your left knee toward the floor. Tilt your pelvis forward until you feel a mild tension in the front of your left hip. Hold for a cycle of relaxation breathing then return to an upright position and reverse. Be sure not to let your front knee bend too far forward. It should remain stacked over your ankle to avoid excess pressure on the knee.

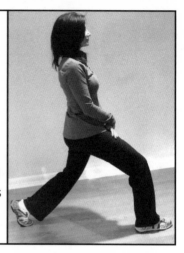

Overhead Stretch

Stand straight and tall with your arms extended overhead. Clasp your hands and inhale as you stretch as high as possible. Exhale as you gently lean your torso to the side. Inhale and return to center, then exhale and lean to the other side.

Try not to let your back arch or your chest push forward. Your movement should be only straight up and to the side.

Variation 1:
Perform the stretch while holding a band or towel.

Variation 2:
Cross your right hand over the left and bend to the side. You will feel a stretch along your entire side. Reverse by crossing your left hand over the right.

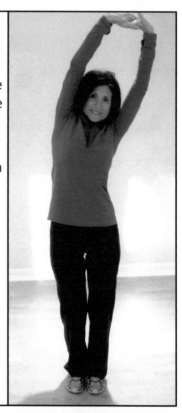

Weight Shift

Stand with your legs in a wide stance and your toes turned out. Shift your weight over your right knee, bending that knee and keeping your left leg straight. Extend your right arm to the side and carry your left arm across your body (shown). To reverse, slowly shift your weight to your left side and swing your arms across your body so they change sides as well. Continue to shift your weight from right to left, ensuring a fluid motion and deepening the stretch with each shift.

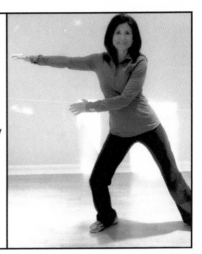

Frisbee Throw

In a wide stance, begin by bending one knee and leaning slightly toward it. Imagine you are holding a Frisbee in the opposite hand, and it is resting near the thigh of your bent leg. Shift your weight to the opposite knee while simultaneously

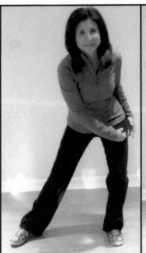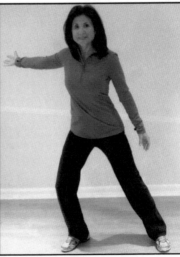

"throwing" your Frisbee by opening that arm to the side and reaching slightly behind you. Continue shifting weight from side to side, reaching a bit farther back each time you repeat the stretch. Reverse.

Remember: Control the movement slowly and smoothly.

Chapter 13

Total Body Stretching: Floor

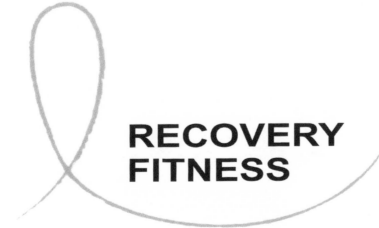

RECOVERY FITNESS

Total Body Stretching: Floor

To aid with comfort in the floor stretches, lie on a mat or a towel. Yoga mats work particularly well. If you have just recently undergone surgery, and are not yet comfortable getting down and up from the floor, these stretches may be performed lying on your bed. A firmer mattress will be helpful for back support. Please note that twisting stretches are contraindicated for osteoporosis.

Floor Stretches without Equipment

Stretching Rack

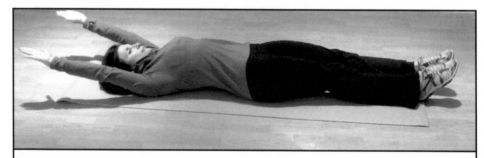

Lie flat on your back with your legs fully extended in front of you, and your arms fully extended overhead. Imagine that someone is pulling on your feet and on your hands at the same time, stretching them as far from the center of your body as possible. Reach as far as you can, then hold the stretch through two cycles of relaxation breathing: breathe in for 5 seconds, breathe out for 5 seconds, repeat. This lengthening stretch will help with opening up the spaces between your vertebrae to decompress your spine and take pressure off your lower back. You will also be stretching areas that may have a build-up of scar tissue. This stretch will assist with the softening and breaking down of that scar tissue as well.

Butterfly Arms

Lie flat on your back with your knees bent and your feet flat on the floor. Bring your hands behind your head with your elbows flat against the floor. Slowly fold your elbows up toward each other. Inhale for 5 seconds as you lift your elbows. Exhale for 5 seconds as you lower your elbows back to the floor to their opened starting position.

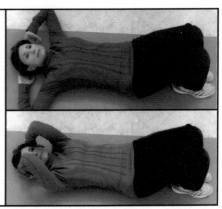

Snow Angels

Lie flat on your back with your arms at your sides. Slowly slide your arms upward over your head. Slowly slide your arms back down to your sides and repeat.

Variation: This stretch may be done standing with your back against a wall.

Knee Drops

Lie flat on your back with your knees bent and your feet flat on the floor. Bring your hands behind your head with your elbows flat against the floor. Pull your knees toward your chest, then slowly drop your knees over to one side while maintaining the position of your upper body. Hold this stretch through a cycle of relaxation breathing, then bring your knees back to center and reverse. Only lower your knees as far as they can go to one side without twisting your lower back off the floor.

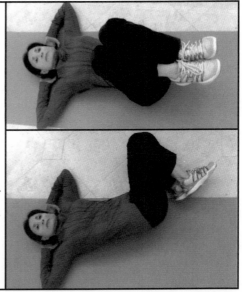

Shoulder Opener

Lie on one side with your knees bent to hip level and stacked one on top of the other. Reach both arms out in front of your chest, with one arm stacked on top of the other. Slowly open the top arm toward the ceiling and continue to open it as you rotate your torso to the opposite side. End with both arms open to the sides and your upper body as open as possible while maintaining the original position of your hips and legs. Hold the stretch through a cycle of relaxation breathing, then return to the starting position and reverse. You may not be able to open up all the way at first, but your goal is to increase your range of motion with each stretch, and eventually have both shoulder blades touching the floor in the open position.

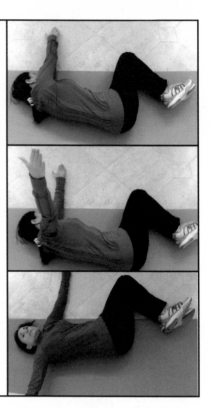

Torso Stretch

Lie flat on your back with your legs extended and arms open to the side. Slowly lift one leg toward the ceiling until it is perpendicular, then lower it across your body toward the floor (shown). Hold the stretch through a cycle of relaxation breathing, then slowly raise the extended leg back toward the ceiling, lower it back to its starting position, and reverse. Try to keep your upper body still throughout the stretch and press your shoulder blades to the floor.

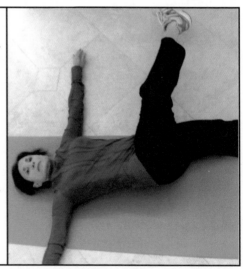

Supine Rotator Cuff Stretch

Lie on your back with your knees bent and your feet flat on the floor. Bring your arms out to the side, then bend your elbows so that your forearms are perpendicular to the floor with your palms facing forward and fingertips pointing toward the ceiling (shown in 1). Pull your shoulder blades down and back without increasing the arch in your lower back or lifting your ribs or hips off the floor. Gently rotate your right forearm backward toward the floor while rotating your left forearm forward toward the floor (2). Your goal is to rotate your forearms until the forearms, wrists and hands all make contact with the floor and are aligned together. Hold the stretch through a cycle of relaxation breathing before slowly returning to your starting position. Reverse the stretch by rotating your left forearm backward toward the floor while rotating your right forearm forward toward the floor (3).

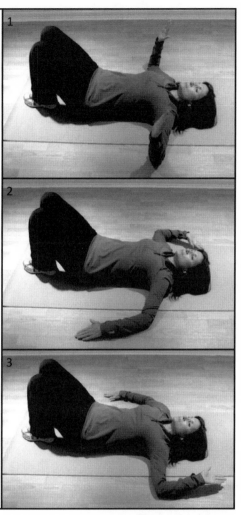

Supine Leg Stretch

This stretch works your lower back, hamstring, calf, and ankle. Lie on your back with your knees bent and your feet flat on the floor. Bend one knee and hug it into the body. Unfold that leg up toward the ceiling, straightening it and pulling it into the body until tension is felt behind the leg. Point and flex the foot three times and perform three ankle circles in each direction. Lower the leg and repeat with the opposite leg.

Child's Pose

Kneel on the floor, then sit on your heels and separate your knees about as wide as your hips while keeping your toes touching together. Lean your belly down between your thighs and reach your arms straight out in front of you, simultaneously pulling your arms and hips in opposite directions. Press your hands in to the floor and hold the stretch through at least one cycle of relaxation breathing. Slide your hands out to a wider position and hold this stretch through at least one cycle of relaxation breathing.

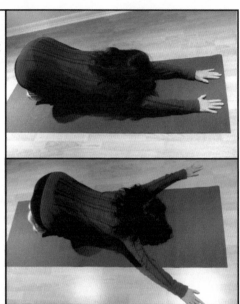

Variation: Child's Pose with Lateral Flexion

Perform the Child's Pose stretch above, but after you lean your belly down between your thighs and reach your arms straight out in front of you, walk your hands to the right until your feel a stretch in your left side; reverse.

Cow/Cat Stretch

Begin on your hands and knees in a table-top position. Make sure your knees are directly below your hips, and that your wrists, elbows and shoulders are in line with each other. As you inhale, lift your chest toward the ceiling, press your belly toward the floor and lift your head. As you exhale, round your spine toward the ceiling and lower your head toward the floor. Repeat each movement 5-10 times with slow and controlled breathing.

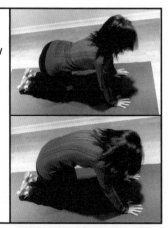

Seated Butterfly Stretch

Sit up tall with the soles of your feet pressed together and your knees dropped to the sides as far as is comfortable. Pull your abdominals gently inward and lean forward from your hips. Holding your ankles, gently pull yourself farther forward. You should feel a stretch in your inner thighs, the outermost part of your hips, and lower back. Increase the intensity by moving your feet toward your body and/or by pressing your thighs toward the floor as you hold the stretch. To reduce stress on your knees, move your feet away from your body.

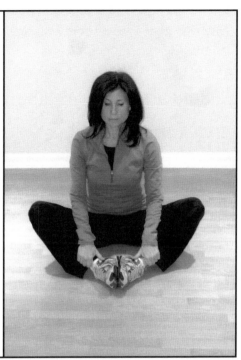

Seated Hip Stretch

Sit up tall, extending your left leg straight out in front of you. Cross your right leg over the left and place your foot on the floor next to the outside of your left knee. Rotate your torso to the right so that the front of your body is facing away from the extended leg, and wrap your left arm around your bent leg (shown). Gently pull against your bent leg to increase the stretch and rotation. Hold the stretch through a cycle of relaxation breathing, then reverse.

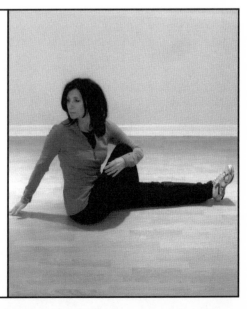

Floor Stretches with Band/Towel

These stretches are performed using a flat resistance band or a towel while sitting or lying on the floor. Using the band or towel allows your stronger side to assist your weaker side as you gain flexibility.

Shoulder Flexion Variations

Standard Grip

Lie flat on your back, bend your knees and place your feet flat on the floor. Hold a flat resistance band or a towel in both hands and begin with your arms lowered to your sides. Slowly lift your arms toward the ceiling and continue to carry them as far back as you are able without causing pain. Hold the stretch at the top for a cycle of relaxation breathing, then lower your arms.

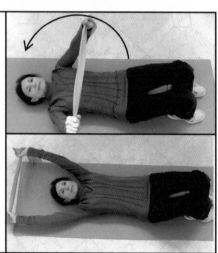

Wide Grip

Perform the shoulder flexion stretch shown above, but with a wider grip on the resistance band or towel (hold a longer length of the band between your hands).

Ball in Place of Band

Perform the shoulder flexion stretch shown above, but hold a large exercise ball in place of the band. Begin with the ball lowered to your stomach. Raise the ball overhead, keeping your elbows straight. Once the ball is overhead, reach with straight arms to the left and then to the right. Return the ball to center and slowly lower it to your starting position.

Shoulder and Torso Stretch Variations

Side Arm

Lie on your back with your arms reaching up toward the ceiling, holding a flat resistance band between both hands. Reach your arms across your chest to the left at shoulder height and drop your knees to the right to roll on to your right hip (shown). Hold the stretch for 10-30 seconds, then return to your starting position and reverse by reaching your arms to the right as you drop your knees to the left.

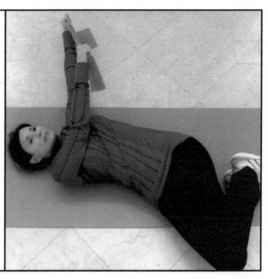

Diagonal Arm

Lie on your back with your arms reaching up toward the ceiling, holding a flat resistance band between both hands. Reach your arms over your left shoulder and drop your knees to the right to roll on to your right hip (shown). Hold the stretch for 10-30 seconds, then return to your starting position and reverse by reaching your arms over your right shoulder as you drop your knees to the left.

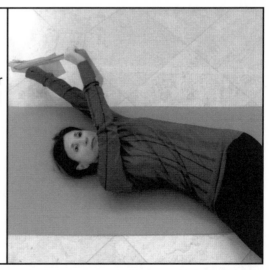

Tip: Do not pull or stretch the band/towel during these exercises. It is simply used to maintain your arm spacing during the stretches.

Floor Stretches with Foam Roller

Lying on a foam roller or large rolled up towel or blanket can allow gravity to assist in increasing your flexibility and range of motion. The following stretches focus on upper body motion, but you will also be using your core muscles to stabilize your body on top of the foam roller.

Pectoral Stretch with Foam Roller

Lie on your back on top of the foam roller. Bend your knees and place your feet flat on the floor. Inhale while bringing your arms up toward the ceiling, palms together at the top. Exhale while opening your arms out to the side until you feel tension in the stretch, but not pain. Your arms may extend slightly behind your shoulders. Hold your arms in the open position through a cycle of relaxation breathing, then bring your arms back up to the starting position.

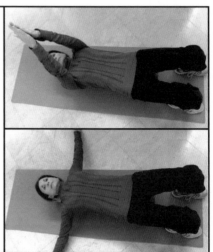

Arm Circles with Foam Roller

Lie on your back on top of the foam roller with your knees bent and your feet flat on the floor. Circle your arms. Start small and gradually increase the size of each circle.

Overhead Stretch with Foam Roller

Open your arms overhead with your elbows at ear level, and gently press your arms toward the floor. Hold your arms in this position through a cycle of relaxation breathing, then bring your arms back up to the starting position.

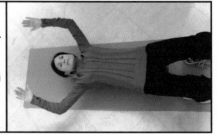

Y Stretch with Foam Roller

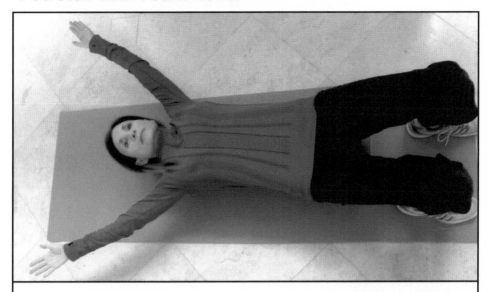

Lie on your back on top of the foam roller with your knees bent and your feet flat on the floor. Open your arms on a diagonal to form the letter Y and gently press your arms toward the floor. Hold this position through a cycle of relaxation breathing, then bring your arms to the starting position.

W Stretch with Foam Roller

Lie on your back on top of the foam roller with your knees bent and your feet flat on the floor. Position your arms overhead in full shoulder flexion, then slowly pull your elbows down and back as if sliding them into your back pockets. Your arms will form a W shape. Hold your arms in this position through a cycle of relaxation breathing, then bring your arms back up to the starting position.

T-Y Stretch with Foam Roller

Lie on your back on top of the foam roller with your knees bent and your feet flat on the floor. Position your arms opened out to the sides, forming the letter T. Slowly carry your arms up to form the letter Y, then carry them back to your sides and repeat.

Stretches with Large Exercise Ball

Using the ball allows for a greater range of motion when lying on your back (similar to using the foam roller), and also helps strengthen your core as you work to maintain your balance on the ball during the stretches.

Pectoral Stretching on the Ball

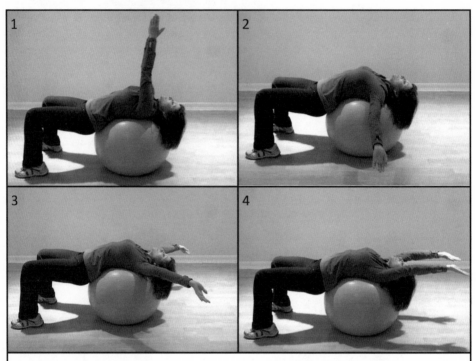

Lie with your back on the ball and your feet flat on the floor in front of you, knees bent at a 90° angle. Raise your arms up with your palms facing each other and your fingertips pointed toward the ceiling (shown in 1). Slowly open your arms out to the side (2), allowing your arms to hang down past your shoulders to open up the chest and achieve a deeper stretch. Hold for a cycle of relaxation breathing, then slowly carry your arms backward to form a Y shape (3) with your palms facing upward. Hold for a cycle of relaxation breathing, then continue to carry your arms backward until they are reaching directly behind your head (4) and hold.

Variation: Rather than holding specific arm positions, make continuous arm circles. Try to increase the size of the circles with each rep.

Butterfly Stretch on the Ball

Lie with your back on the ball and your feet flat on the floor in front of you, knees bent at a 90° angle. Open your elbows out to the side and place your fingertips behind your head. Allow gravity to pull your shoulders down and hold the stretch for a cycle of relaxation breathing.

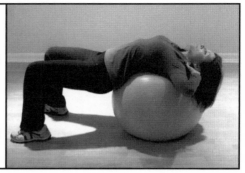

Child's Pose on the Ball

Kneel in front of the ball. Place both hands on the top of the ball and roll the ball forward away from your body (do not move your knees). Roll the ball back to the starting position. Then roll the ball to the left, and back to the starting position, then to the right, and back to the starting position.

Side Stretch on the Ball

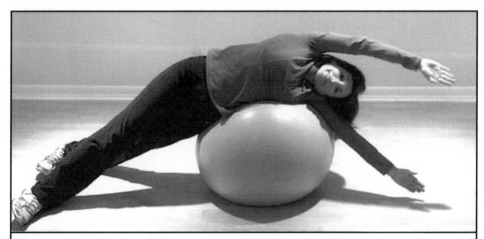

Drape one side over the ball with your legs straight and your top leg slightly in front of your bottom leg to assist with balance. Extend your arms overhead with your palms facing forward. Allow gravity to deepen your side stretch. Hold for a cycle of relaxation breathing, then turn to the other side and repeat the stretch.

Chapter 14

Strengthening

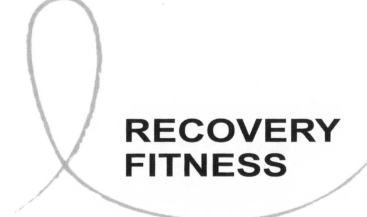

RECOVERY FITNESS

Strengthening

Move gently when performing strength training exercises, allowing for slow and progressive improvement. Control and good form are essential. Perform only as many repetitions as possible while controlling the movement and maintaining good form. You may want to use a mirror or a partner to help you achieve proper form if you are not familiar with the exercises.

Floor Exercises

To aid with comfort, lie on a mat or a towel during these strengthening exercises. Yoga mats work particularly well. Many of these exercises can be done in bed if you are not able to do floor exercises yet.

Pelvic Tilt

Lie on your back with your knees bent and your feet flat on the floor. Inhale and fill your torso with air. Exhale while pressing your abdominals downward, bringing your navel to your spine. Lower and repeat for 5-10 reps.

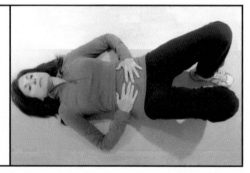

Pelvic Tilt with Kegels

Lie on your back with your knees bent and your feet flat on the floor. Inhale and fill your torso with air. Exhale while pressing your abdominals downward, bringing your navel to your spine. While in the tilt position, add Kegels: Squeeze the pelvic floor muscles for 5 seconds, then release. Lower your pelvis and repeat the exercise for 5-10 reps.
Note: You can find your pelvic floor muscles by squeezing your sphincter and contracting the urethra as if trying to stop the flow of urination. The muscles used to stop the flow of urine are the pelvic floor muscles.

Bridge

Lie on your back with your knees bent and your feet flat on the floor. Squeeze your glutes to lift your pelvis and ribs off the ground, leaving only your shoulders on the floor. Hold the bridge position for a few seconds, then lower and repeat. Complete 5-10 reps.

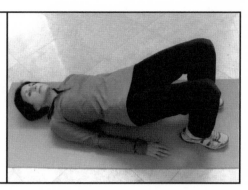

One Leg Bridge

Lie on your back with your knees bent and your feet flat on the floor. Squeeze your glutes to lift your pelvis and ribs off the ground, leaving only your shoulders on the floor. Lift one leg up to the ceiling and hold for a few seconds. Lower your leg, lower your body, and repeat the exercise lifting the opposite leg.

Bridge with Towel/Ball

Lie on your back with your knees bent and your feet flat on the floor. Place a towel or a small ball between your knees. Squeeze your glutes to lift your pelvis and ribs off the ground, leaving only your shoulders on the floor. Hold the bridge position as you squeeze the towel 8 times, then lower and repeat for 5-10 reps.

Leg Slides

Lie on your back with your knees bent and your feet flat on the floor. Inhale to start, then exhale as you slide one leg down to the floor. Inhale as you slide the leg back to its starting position. Repeat on the other leg. Complete 5-10 reps with each leg.

Hip Strengthener

Lie on your side with your bottom arm tucked underneath your head for support and your top arm resting in front of your body. Bend your knees and pull them up toward your chest so that your thighs and torso form a 90° angle. Keep your legs and feet stacked directly on top of each other. This is your starting position. Lift your top leg about 10 inches, then lower and repeat. Perform 5-10 reps then reverse lying on your opposite side. When lifting your leg, try to maintain its position parallel to your resting leg; do not let either your knee or your ankle drop.

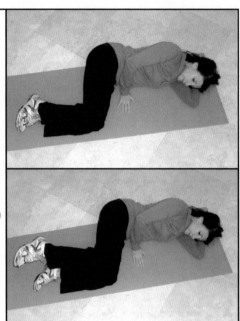

Clamshell Exercise

Lie on your side with your bottom arm tucked underneath your head for support and your top arm resting in front of your body. Bend your knees and pull them up toward your chest so that your thighs and torso form a 90° angle. Keep your legs and feet stacked directly on top of each other. This is your starting position. Keeping your ankles in place, rotate your hip to lift your top knee toward the ceiling. Perform 5-10 reps then reverse lying on your opposite side.

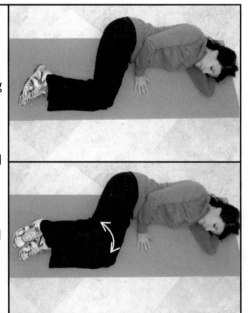

Superman Core Exercise

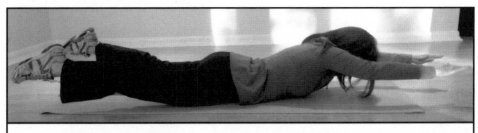

Lie face down on the floor and extend your arms straight out in front of you. Use your lower back muscles to lift your chest and arms slightly off the floor while simultaneously lifting your legs slightly off the floor. Contract your glutes and hold the position for 5 seconds, then relax and lower your chest, arms and legs to the floor. Repeat 5-10 times.

Alternating Superman

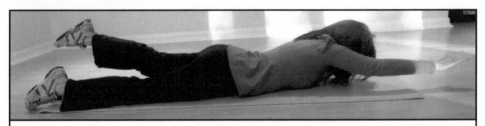

Lie face down on the floor and extend your arms straight out in front of you. Lift one arm and the opposite leg slightly off the floor, keeping your head in line with your spine. Hold for 5 seconds then lower and reverse.

Superman with Scapular Retraction

Perform the Superman exercise above and when your arms are lifted, bend your elbows and pull back with your upper back and shoulders until your arms form a W. Hold for 5 seconds then lower.

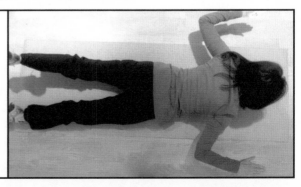

Bird Dog Exercise

Begin on your hands and knees in a table-top position. Make sure your knees are set directly below your hips, that your wrists, elbows and shoulders are in line with each other, and your head is in a neutral position. Contract your abdominals to maintain your balance while you slowly extend one leg directly behind you and simultaneously extend the opposite arm out in front (1). Hold for 10 seconds, then return to table-top position and reverse. When your balance is ready for a challenge, perform the exercise as described, then carry the extended arm out to the side (2) and then back to the front before returning to table-top position.

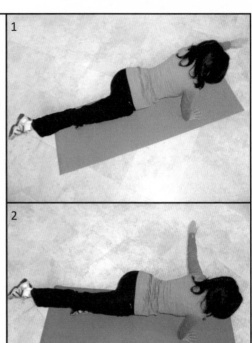

Note: Your core muscles include your abdominals and your back. Strengthening these muscles will help you maintain and improve your balance and improve your posture. Good balance and posture will enhance your ability to perform activities of daily living. Cancer survivors may develop balance and posture issues. The exercises in this book will help to improve poor posture and balance.

Some of the core work used in this program is Pilates based. Pilates focuses on the transverse abdominus, the deepest layer of abdominal muscle, which is why it is so effective in strengthening the core. The deep breathing, concentration and focus keep the core muscles engaged. Each exercise is performed slowly and with control, eliminating momentum. The body is always square to the mat without moving or rocking.

Bird Dog Variations

These exercises build on the basic Bird Dog and provide a greater challenge. Begin on your hands and knees in a table-top position. Make sure your knees are set directly below your hips, that your wrists, elbows and shoulders are in line with each other, and your head is in a neutral position. Contract your abdominals to maintain your balance while you slowly inhale and pull one knee in toward your chest and round your spine toward the ceiling (1). Exhale as you extend your leg directly behind you and release your spine to its neutral position (2). Hold for 10 seconds, then return to table-top position and reverse. When you are ready for more of a challenge, you may add an arm movement. Contract your abdominals to maintain your balance while you slowly inhale and pull one knee in toward your chest, pull your opposite elbow in toward the raised knee, and round your spine toward the ceiling (3). Exhale as you extend your leg directly behind you while simultaneously extending your opposite arm out in front and releasing your spine to its neutral position (4). Hold for 10 seconds, then return to table-top position and reverse.

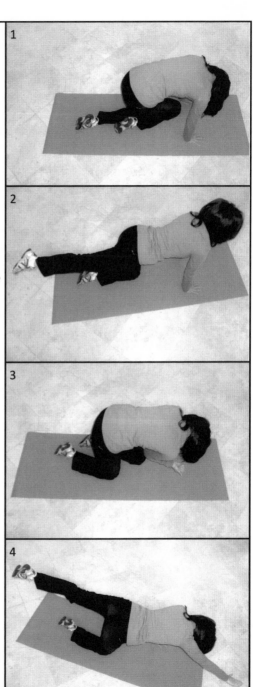

Cross-Over Crunch

Lie flat on your back with your knees bent and your feet flat on the floor. Cross your left ankle over your right knee, bring your right hand behind your head, and leave your left arm down at your side. This is your starting position. Keeping your lower back pressed into the floor, contract your abdominals, lift your shoulder blades off the floor and curl your upper body diagonally across towards your left knee. Return to your starting position. Repeat 5-10 times, then reverse. Be careful not to pull on your neck. The movement should initiate from your core.

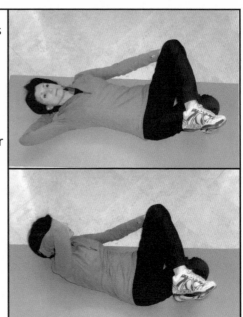

Lateral Crunch

Lie flat on your back with your knees bent and your feet flat on the floor. Bring your right hand behind your head, and leave your left arm down at your side. This is your starting position. Keeping your lower back pressed into the floor, contract your abdominals, lift your shoulder blades slightly off the floor and reach your left arm down towards your left ankle. Return to your starting position. Repeat 5-10 times, then reverse. Be careful not to pull on your neck. The movement should initiate from your core.

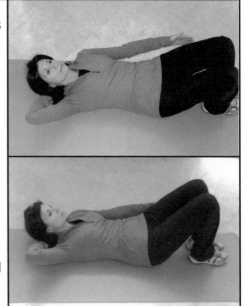

Bicycle Exercise

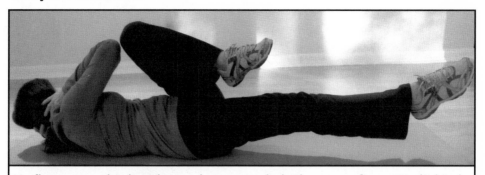

Lie flat on your back with your legs extended. Place your fingertips behind your ears. Contract your abdominals and raise your legs slightly off the ground, then pull one knee in toward your chest while twisting your torso to bring your opposite elbow toward the lifted knee. Reverse. Do not let your legs touch the floor until you are finished with your repetitions.

Side Knee Drops

Lie flat on your back with your arms extended out to the sides and your knees lifted to form a 90° angle. Contract your abdominals and slowly lower your knees to one side until they almost touch the floor. Do not let your knees rest on the floor; keep them lifted a few inches. Slowly raise your knees back to center and reverse. You may not be able to drop your knees all the way to the side at first. Drop them only as far as you are able to hold them steadily and keep your back on the floor. As your abdominals gain strength, you will be able to drop your knees lower toward the floor and be able to lift them back up again.

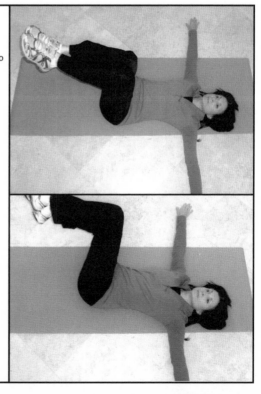

Leg Raises

Lie flat on your back with your arms at your sides and your legs extended up toward the ceiling. Slowly lower your legs toward the floor without arching your back. Do not let your feet touch the floor. Slowly raise your legs back to your starting position and repeat. Keep your movement slow and controlled. If you feel too much pressure on your lower back, you may place your hands underneath your bottom.

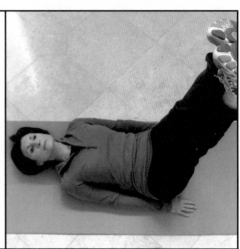

Dead Bug Exercise

Lie flat on your back with your arms and legs extended up toward the ceiling. Inhale as you lower one leg and the opposite arm toward the floor, dropping your leg only as far as you can without letting it touch the floor. Exhale as you raise your arm and leg back to your starting position and reverse. Keep your abdominals engaged throughout the exercise and control your movement. When your arms and legs are working at the same time, your lower back and/or ribs may start to curve up off the floor. Be aware of this and make sure you are pressing your lower back in to the floor throughout the exercise. As your abdominals become stronger, this will become second nature.

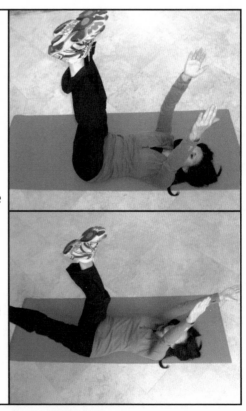

Single Leg Circles

Lie flat on your back with your arms at your sides, knees bent and feet flat on the floor. Raise one leg up toward the ceiling. This is your starting position. Contract your abdominals to keep your body stable while you make small circles in the air with the raised leg. Keep your torso as still as possible. Try to perform 10 circles clockwise and 10 circles counterclockwise, then lower your leg and reverse.

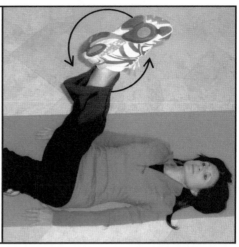

Corkscrew Exercise

Lie flat on your back with your arms at your sides and your legs extended up toward the ceiling. Contract your abdominals to keep your body stable while you make small circles in the air with both legs. Keep your torso as still as possible. Try to perform 10 circles clockwise and 10 circles counterclockwise.

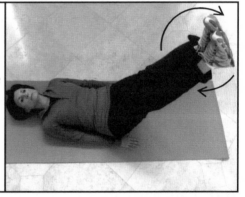

Note: Pilates is a gentle restorative exercise regime, which helps one recover and rebuild. It strengthens and stretches the body. Control, precision, body mechanics and breathing are emphasized. Pilates is non-impact exercise that can help patients regain physical and emotional health. Muscles are strengthened while breathing deeply. It is a great choice for people with, or at risk for, lymphedema. Form is emphasized and it is low repetition: quality over quantity. The workout can be modified to accommodate all fitness levels and issues.

Standing Exercises without Equipment

Calf Raises

Stand up straight with your feet hip-width apart. Slowly raise your heels until you are standing on the balls of your feet. Pause, then slowly lower your heels back down to the floor and repeat. Keep your abdominals engaged to assist with balance. Perform 5-10 reps.

Variation: To increase the intensity, you may hold a light dumbbell in each hand while performing the calf raises.

Note: If you are unable to balance without assistance, you may hold gently on to the back of a chair, or face sideways to a wall and place one hand on the wall for balance.

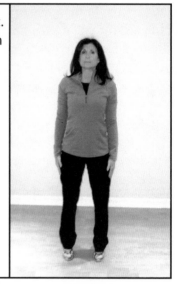

Wall Sit

Place your back and arms against the wall, feet hip-width apart, a foot or two away from the wall. Keeping your back against the wall, lower your hips until your knees form a 90° angle (shown). Hold the position for 30 seconds, then use your hands to slowly walk your body back up the wall to a standing position. If you have knee issues, modify by lowering just a few inches. You may not be able to hold the position for 30 seconds at first. Simply hold as long as you are able, gradually increasing your time with each exercise session. Once you are able to hold the position for 30 seconds with ease, build up to holding the wall sit for up to two minutes.

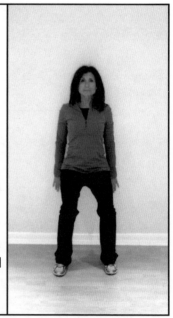

Balance Tree Pose

Stand up straight with your feet close to each other. Place your left foot on your right calf and lift your arms up. Engage your abdominals as you hold this balance pose for 10 seconds. Lower your arms and leg and repeat with the opposite leg.

Knee Lift Balance Pose

Stand up straight with your feet slightly apart. Lift your left knee up for 10 seconds while balancing on your right leg, then switch legs. Your knee does not have to rise very high for this to be an effective balance strengthener. Even lifting your foot just a few inches off the floor will help.

Wall Push-Up

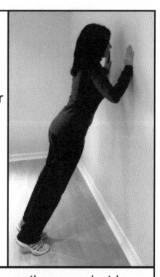

Stand in front of a wall and lift your arms to shoulder level. Place your palms on the wall slightly wider than shoulder-width apart. Back your feet away from the wall and lean on an angle in to the wall (shown). Exhale as you push off the wall until your arms are straight, then inhale and come back to your starting position. Do not arch your back during this exercise. Perform 5-10 reps.

Note: Try to recruit the serratus, the muscle over your ribs on each side below the pectoral chest muscle, which can be involved in winged scapula and needs to be strengthened. Do this by retracting and protracting the scapula in the wall push-up position. Winged scapula occurs when the shoulder blade or bone protrudes, giving a wing-like appearance on the back. It can seriously interfere with activities of daily living, so this is an important strengthening exercise.

Exercises with a Chair

Leg Lifts: Front

Stand with your side to a chair or couch back and rest your inside hand on the chair back for balance. Standing straight and tall, lift your outside leg up to the front to a 45° angle, then slowly lower and repeat. Perform 5-10 reps then switch legs. When you are lifting your leg, try to maintain your body position: do not lean in toward the chair or lean back away from the working leg. Keep your abdominals engaged to maintain your body position and balance. Lift only as high as you can while maintaining good form.

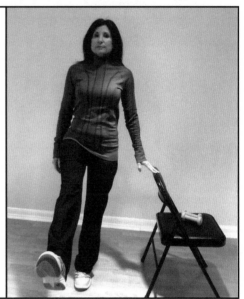

Leg Lifts: Side

Stand with your side to a chair or couch back and rest your inside hand on the chair back for balance. Standing straight and tall, lift your outside leg up to the side to a 45° angle, then slowly lower and repeat. Perform 5-10 reps then switch legs. When you are lifting your leg, try to maintain your body position: do not lean in toward the chair or lean back away from the working leg. Keep your abdominals engaged to maintain your body position and balance. Lift only as high as you can while maintaining good form.

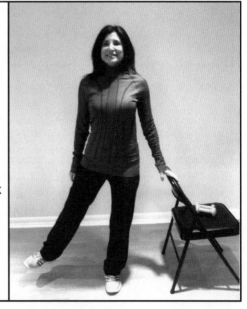

Leg Lifts: Back

Stand facing a chair or couch back and rest your hands on the chair back for balance. Standing straight and tall, lift one leg up behind you to a 45° angle, then slowly lower and repeat. Perform 5-10 reps then switch legs. When you are lifting your leg, you may lean slightly forward (hinge from the hips), but do not lean heavily on the chair. If you lean forward, maintain a straight back; do not let your back or shoulders round forward. Keep your abdominals engaged throughout the exercise to maintain your body's position and balance.

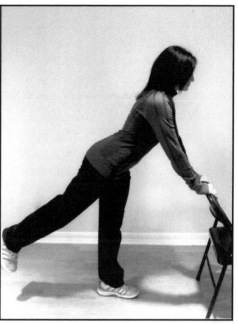

Leg Lifts: Back with Front Reach

Perform the back leg lift exercise above. When you lift your leg, simultaneously raise the opposite arm to the front. Reach your arm and leg as far away from the center of your body as possible. Perform 5-10 reps then switch legs, or perform one rep at a time, alternating sides between each lift. When you are lifting your leg and arm, you may lean slightly forward (hinge from the hips), but do not lean heavily on the chair. If you lean forward, maintain a straight back; do not let your back or shoulders round forward. Keep your abdominals engaged.

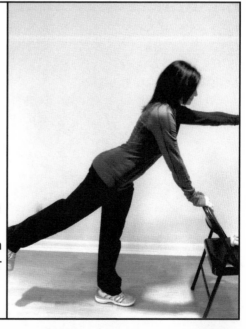

Squats

Stand in front of a chair or couch with your legs hip-width apart, facing away from the chair. Place one hand on your stomach and the other hand on your lower back. Your hands will help you remember to keep your back straight and your abdominals engaged. Slowly bend your knees and lower your bottom backward, as if starting to sit in to the chair. Do not actually sit down. Lower as far as you can, then stand back up and repeat for 5-10 reps.

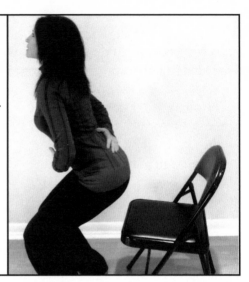

Squats with Hammer Curl

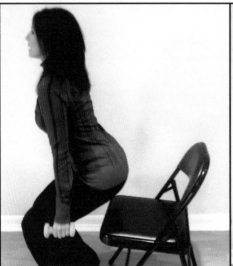
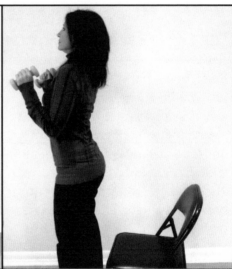

Perform the squat exercise above while holding dumbbells in each hand. Hold the weights with their ends facing forward. As you squat down, inhale and lower your arms to your sides. As you stand back up, exhale and bend your elbows to curl the weights up to your chest. Repeat for 5-10 reps. The compound exercise saves time in your workout session.

Forward Lunges

Stand with your side to a chair or couch back. Place your inside hand on the chair back for support and balance. Step forward with your outside leg and shift your weight on to that leg. Lower your front knee until your thigh is parallel to the floor (shown). Be sure that your knee does not push forward past your ankle. Press up with your legs to return to a straight standing position and repeat for 5-10 reps, then reverse.

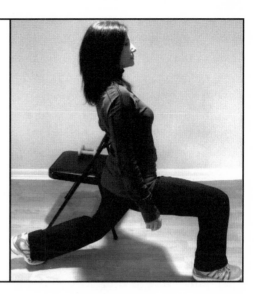

Lunges with Shoulder Press

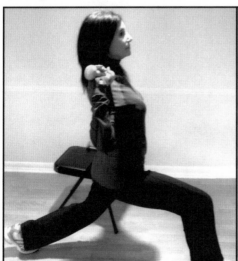

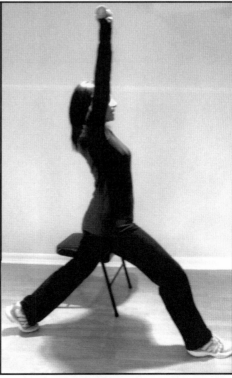

Perform the lunge exercise above while holding dumbbells in each hand. As you lunge down, inhale and hold the weights at shoulder height. As you stand up, exhale and press the weights straight up overhead.

Bent Over Row

Place your left knee and left arm on a chair with your back parallel to the floor, hinged forward from the hips. Hold a dumbbell in your right hand with that arm extended down toward the floor. Exhale as you bend your elbow and lift the weight toward your waist. Inhale as you lower the weight back toward the floor. Repeat for 5-10 reps then switch arms. When lifting the weight, try not to focus solely on your arm. Initiate the movement from your back and shoulders, with the arm movement being secondary. Keep your back straight and your abdominals engaged throughout the exercise, being sure not to round your back or shoulders.

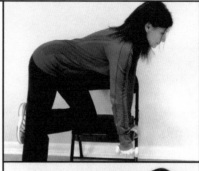
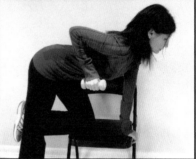

Reverse Fly

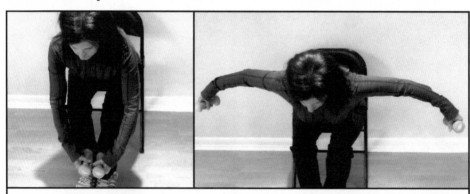

Sit in a chair holding a dumbbell in each hand. Hinge forward from the hips until your chest is close to your thighs and your arms are extended down toward the floor. Keeping your arms slightly bent, slowly raise the weights up and out to the sides. Raise them as high as they can go and squeeze your shoulder blades together. Pause at the top of the movement, then slowly lower the weights back to the starting position. Perform 5-10 reps.

Floor Exercises with Free Weights

Supine Protraction Chest Press

Note: This exercise may be performed lying on a bench, on the floor, or on a large exercise ball. Start with no weight (positioning your hands as if they were holding dumbbells), and gradually add weight.

Lie flat on your back with your knees bent and your feet flat on the floor. Hold a dumbbell in each hand if you are using weight. Push the dumbbells up so that your arms are directly over your shoulders. Contract your abdominals and tilt your chin slightly toward your chest. This is your starting position. Inhale as you lower the dumbbells down toward your chest. Roll your shoulder blades back and down, as if you are pinching them together and accentuating your chest. Exhale as you push the weights back up, taking care not to lock your elbows or allow your shoulder blades to rise off the bench/floor/ball. Perform 5-10 reps.

Supine Scapula Protraction

Note: This exercise may be performed lying on a bench, on the floor, or on a large exercise ball.

Lie flat on your back with your knees bent and your feet flat on the floor. Hold a dumbbell in one hand. Push the dumbbell up so that your arm is directly over your shoulder. Contract your abdominals and tilt your chin slightly toward your chest. This is your starting position. Inhale to start, then exhale as you push the weight straight up. Reach as far toward the ceiling as possible by moving your shoulder blade toward the ceiling. Then lower your shoulder blade back to the starting position, keeping your elbow straight. Perform 5-10 reps, then repeat with the opposite arm.

Standing Exercises with Free Weights

Biceps Curl

Stand with a dumbbell in each hand, arms extended down toward the floor, palms facing forward. Exhale as you bend your elbows and curl the weights up toward your shoulders. Inhale as you slowly straighten your arms and return to your starting position. Perform 5-10 reps.

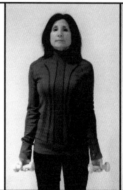 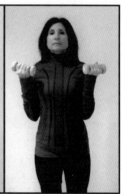

Lateral Arm Raises

Stand with a dumbbell in each hand, palms facing in toward your sides. Inhale to start, then exhale as you raise your right arm out to the side, stopping when your elbow reaches shoulder height. Keep your arm straight, but don't lock the elbow, and keep your palm facing down during the raise. Inhale as you slowly lower your hand back to your side. You should be able to see your hand in your peripheral vision during the raise, so your arm is slightly forward, not directly out to the side. Perform 5-10 reps with the right arm, the left arm, and with both arms simultaneously.

Overhead Triceps Extension

Stand with a dumbbell in each hand, arms extended up toward the ceiling, palms facing each other. Inhale as you bend your elbows and lower the weights down behind your head. Exhale as you unfold and extend your arms back up to your starting position. Perform 5-10 reps.

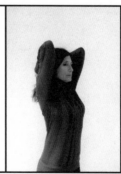 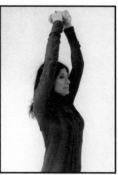

Shoulder Flexion

Stand with a dumbbell in each hand, arms extended down toward the floor, palms facing back. Inhale to start, then exhale as you raise your right arm in front of your body, stopping when your elbow reaches shoulder height. Keep your arm straight, but don't lock the elbow, and keep your palm facing down during the raise. Inhale as you slowly lower your arm back to the starting position. Perform 5-10 reps with the right arm, the left arm, and with both arms simultaneously.

Shoulder Press

Stand with a dumbbell in each hand, elbows bent, hands at shoulder-level, palms facing forward. Exhale as you press the weights up toward the ceiling, extending your arms overhead. Inhale as you slowly lower your arms and return to your starting position. Perform 5-10 reps.

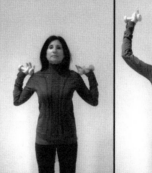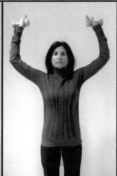

Scaption

Stand with a dumbbell in each hand, arms extended down toward the floor, palms facing in toward your sides. Inhale to start, then exhale as you raise your arms at an angle in front of your body (so that they form a "Y"), stopping when your arms are parallel to the floor. Keep your arms straight, but don't lock the elbows. Inhale as you slowly lower your arms back to the starting position. Perform 5-10 reps.

Remember: Be patient. Getting back to your previous fitness level may take time. Track your progress and improve slowly to avoid injury.

Exercises with Resistance Band

Seated Row

Sit up tall on the floor with your legs extended straight out in front of you with a resistance band wrapped around the bottom of both feet. Exhale as you pull your shoulders back, pulling the band back until your hands are next to your waist. Squeeze your shoulder blades together at the back of the row. Inhale as you slowly release your arms forward until they are back in starting position. Perform 5-10 reps.

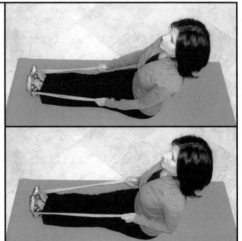

Standing Anchored Row Variations

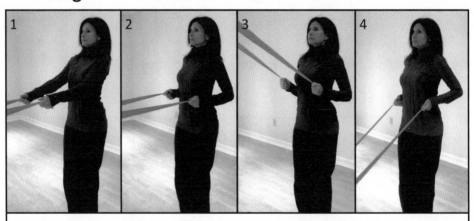

Inexpensive door anchors may be purchased for anchored band exercises. Anchor your resistance band at waist height with your arms extended out in front of you (1). Exhale as you pull your shoulders back, pulling the band back until your hands are next to your waist (2). Squeeze your shoulder blades together at the back of the row. Inhale as you slowly release your arms forward until they are back in starting position. Perform 5-10 reps. Anchor your band high (3) or low (4) for variations on the row.

Rotator Cuff Exercises

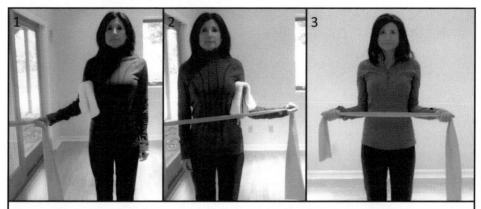

Internal rotation: Anchor your band at waist level and stand sideways to the band, holding it in your inside hand with your elbow bent at your side (shown in 1). Exhale as you rotate your arm to bring the band across your waist, keeping your elbow in place. Inhale as you open your arm and return the band to the starting position. External rotation: Holding the band in your outside hand with your arm folded across your waist, exhale as you rotate your arm to bring your forearm out to the side, keeping your elbow in place (shown in 2). Inhale as you close your arm and return the band to the starting position. Without anchor: Hold your band in both hands, elbows bent, palms facing up and forearms extended in front of you. Exhale as you externally rotate your arms, keeping your elbows in place (shown in 3). Inhale and resist the movement as you return the band to the starting position. Perform 5-10 reps of each exercise on each side.

Lat Pull-Down

Stand with your band in both hands, arms extended up in front of you slightly wider than shoulder-width apart. Exhale as you pull your arms apart and down to waist level. Inhale as you raise them back up.

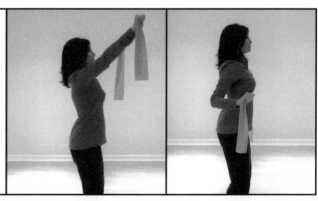

Exercises with Large Exercise Ball

Wall Sit and Arm Circles with Ball

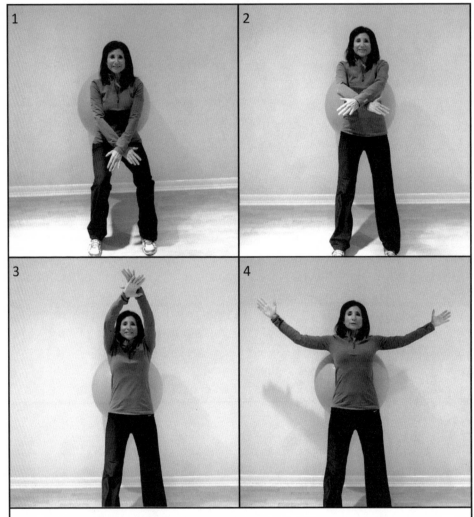

Place your ball behind your back against the wall, feet hip-width apart, arms extended down and crossed in front of your body. Keeping your back against the ball, lower your hips to the starting position (1). Slowly roll your back up the ball to a standing position (2), raise your arms overhead (3), and open them back and around (4) to perform a large arm circle. Return to your starting position and repeat for 5-10 reps.

Plié Wall Sit with Ball

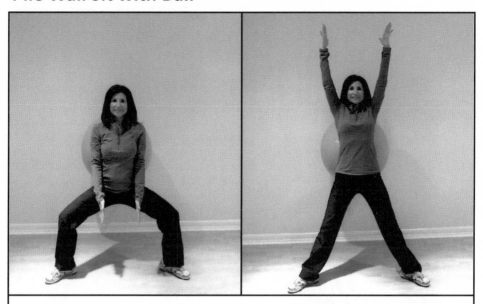

Place your ball behind your back against the wall, feet in a wide second position stance with toes turned out, arms extended straight down in front of your body. Keeping your back against the ball, inhale as you bend your knees into a deep plié. Exhale as you roll your back up against the ball, straightening your legs and carrying your arms up in front of you until they are extended straight overhead. Repeat for 5-10 reps.

Increase the Intensity: Any of the Wall Sits with the large exercise ball can also be performed on your toes. This will add intensity for your leg muscles and challenge your balance as well.

Shoulder Stretching and Strengthening on the Ball

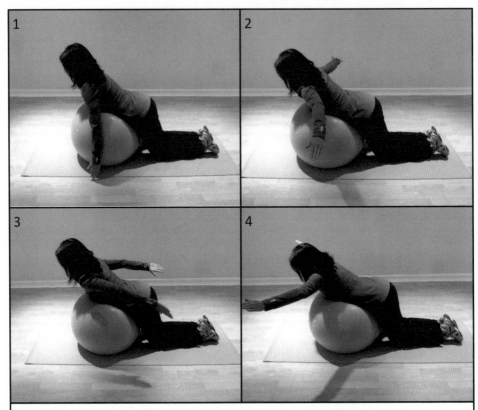

Kneel with the ball in front of you and lean forward, resting your stomach on the ball. Let your arms hang down along the sides of the ball (shown in 1). Slowly open your arms out to the side (2), squeezing your shoulder blades together to initiate the movement. Hold for a cycle of relaxation breathing, then slowly carry your arms behind you (3) with your palms facing upward. Hold for a cycle of relaxation breathing, then rotate your shoulders to turn your palms toward the floor as you slowly carry your arms forward to a Y shape (4). Hold for a cycle of relaxation breathing.

Hand and Foot Exercises

Hand Press

Press your hands together, then press your index fingers away from each other. Press your index fingers back together. Repeat the same motion (press away, press back together) with each finger.

Finger Touch

Open your palm and bring your index finger to your thumb. Release your fingers and repeat the movement of touching one finger to your thumb with each finger. Repeat with the fingers on your opposite hand.

Fist Pump

Close your hand in to a fist, then release. Perform this exercise with your arms up and then with your arms in front of you. Repeat with the opposite hand.

Note: This may help decrease swelling after surgery by using your muscles as a pump. You can perform this exercise while in bed.

Wrist Curls

Hold a light dumbbell in each hand. Bend your elbows by your sides so that your forearms are parallel to the floor and your hands are out in front of your body. With your palms facing down, curl your wrists up and down for 5-10 reps. Repeat the wrist curl with your palms facing up for 5-10 reps. When you have completed the curls, continue to hold your arms in the same position and rotate your palms up and down for 5-10 reps.

Toe Clenching

To help strengthen your feet, clench your toes and then relax them. This can be done standing, sitting, or lying down. Perform 5-10 reps.

Additional Reading

♦ Lymphedema: A Personal Trainer's Perspective

♦ Exercise Tips from "10 to Thrive"

♦ Health Needs of Low Income Communities

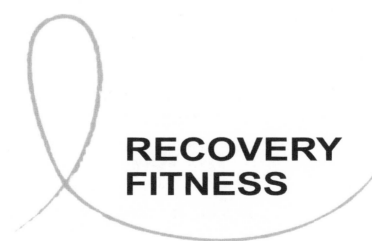

**RECOVERY
FITNESS**

Lymphedema: A Personal Trainer's Perspective

Carol Michaels wrote this article for the National Lymphedema Network, published January/March 2013.

Cancer surgery and treatment often results in survivors suffering debilitating physical impairments. These can often be ameliorated by a good exercise program that has the added benefit of helping survivors to engage in those activities in which they participated prior to their diagnosis. This article addresses some of the physical side effects cancer survivors may face; including lymphedema and a series of safe and effective techniques to restore functional fitness for those with or at risk for lymphedema.

Surgery, chemotherapy, radiation, and hormonal therapy have side effects, which exacerbate the problems faced by cancer patients. Surgery can create adhesions that can limit range of motion, and cause pain, numbness and tightness. Removal of lymph nodes creates scars and may decrease range of motion. Radiation can cause fatigue, tightness and stiffness. It also can increase the risk of developing lymphedema. Chemotherapy may affect balance, a patient's immune system, and cause neuropathy, fatigue, sarcopenia, and anemia. Hormonal therapy can cause joint pain and early menopause and the side effects associated with menopause.

Before beginning a cancer exercise program, a patient must receive medical clearance. A medical history, base line range of motion and girth measurements, and a general fitness assessment are taken. It is important to note that many exercises and movements may be contraindicated based on a person's fitness assessment, medical conditions, and particular surgery. There are different exercises necessary for each type of reconstruction. For those who were active prior to surgery it is imperative to slowly work back up to the previous level of activity. It is not wise to go back to a gym and continue with a pre-cancer exercise routine.

Research has shown that exercise is safe for cancer survivors, even those with or who are at risk for lymphedema. Dr. Schmitz stresses the importance of starting slowly and using proper form with a well trained certified professional. Her study demonstrates the importance of exercise after cancer with slow progressive improvement in order to decrease risk of lymphedema. The research shows that breast cancer survivors no longer have to give up activities that they enjoy doing and avoid activities of daily living. Aerobic exercise is essential to good health and we advise a patient to walk as much as possible. Initially, one might start by walking around their house or up and down their block and then slowly increasing the distance walked. Many physicians recommend that their patients try to walk during chemotherapy. This may decrease fatigue. If using aerobic equipment make sure not to grip on the railing.

Unfortunately, there is no way to know which patients with lymph node dissection will get lymphedema. This makes it imperative to follow the established guidelines and take prudent approach to exercise. Patients who have lymphedema need to progress slowly and use a properly fitted garment. Our goal is to promote physical activity without exacerbating lymphedema. Severe range of motion issues and cording problems are referred to lymphedema specialists. Moreover, measurement of the limbs that are at risk for lymphedema are performed frequently to make sure they have not changed in size. Symptoms can be managed easier if they are addressed promptly. Progress is monitored in order to make appropriate modifications to a patient's program. It is important to learn the right exercises for a patient's particular situation and how to do them properly and with good form. The patient should learn which exercises to perform, the sequencing and quantity. Exercise smartly and under professional guidance!

Lymphedema can be debilitating and painful and can affect the emotional health of the patient. Our bodies work better if engaged in regular physical activity, but it must be done in a safe manner if lymph nodes have been removed or radiated. A cancer fitness program for someone with lymphedema should begin as an individualized program. The patient must be supervised to make sure there are no subtle volume changes to the limb. Ultimately, we want a patient to be able to exercise on his or her own.

The starting point is a low impact exercise program, performing range of motion stretches and techniques to improve venous drainage. First, we elevate the affected area above heart level. Over time, stretches are incorporated until a patient can achieve 80% of range of motion. At that point, we start adding strength training. A stretching program for those with upper body lymphedema begins with moving or stretching the neck and shoulder areas. If a patient is still healing from breast cancer surgery, begin with pendulum arm swings. The arm is then moved and stretched in all directions: going across the chest and behind the head and back. Stretches that move the arms in shoulder flexion, extension, abduction, and adduction are added. Finally internal and external rotations are addressed. Patients suffering from fatigue can perform many of the stretches while in bed. An easy to follow DVD is Recovery Fitness Simple Stretching, which can be found on www.recoveryfitness.net.

All of the exercises incorporate abdominal breathing, which can stimulate lymphatic drainage. This intra-abdominal pressure may help move sluggish lymph fluid, stimulate lymph flow, and act as a lymphatic system pump. This type of breathing enables oxygen to get to the tissues. Abdominal breathing and relaxation breathing, along with the proper exercises can also reduce stress, a common cancer side effect. If weak, it may be best just to stretch and breathe deeply.

Strength training may help pump the lymph fluid away from the affected limb. Exercise helps the lymphatic fluid to move. Muscles pump and push the lymph fluid and can help move the lymph from the affected area. Strength training may also strengthen the arm so that it can handle those activities that may have otherwise led to swelling with a greater level of ease. Always wear a sleeve and stop if there is swelling or pain. Start with light weights and slowly increase repetitions and eventually weight.

Cancer survivors should follow a systematic and progressive plan. Exercise starts with a warm-up and ends with a cool down. Begin with deep breathing. Keeping a strong core should be emphasized. It is important to remember that following treatment the body may have become weaker. Even if a patient had exercised using 10 pound weights before surgery, if one is at risk for lymphedema they must start with a light weight. We teach patients to always listen to their bodies and to stop if they feel tired or if their limb aches or feels heavy. Patients must be aware of any changes in their body.

Progression of exercise should be gradual. A deconditioned person should start without using any weight and concentrate on proper technique. If 8-10 repetitions can not be executed, repetitions should be decreased or the weight lowered or resistance band used changed to less resistance. The exercise routines have to be adapted for the day to day changes that can affect the ability to work out. Our program will start using a very light weight, with few repetitions, typically 10. In subsequent sessions, patients can add repetitions. After performing two sets of 10 repetitions with no problem then a small amount of weight may be added in 1-pound increments. We also alternate between strength training exercises with a stretch for each muscle group and to alternate an upper body and lower body exercises. Pilates exercises are a great way to incorporate deep breathing with strengthening the core. The deep breathing helps to pump lymphatic fluid and will also help reduce stress.

Every patient is unique. Many patients have pre-existing medical issues. The exercise program should be modified to accommodate all body types and needs. Some might need pillows for comfort or postural problems. Also if osteoporosis is an issue, a cancer therapist should have experience working with this population. Always monitor the affected limb. Look for feelings of fullness or aching. We do not want to overwhelm the lymphatic system. Drink plenty of water and stop immediately if any pain. Lymphedema patients should elevate their limbs after a session.

Learn which aerobic exercises are considered safe. Walking, biking, and swimming are considered very safe. Hot tubs, pools, and warm lakes may increase risk of infection. In choosing an activity, consider the risk of injury, prior medical condition, and fitness level. Injuries can create further complications for those with lymphedema. It is still unclear whether certain sports can be safe. For example, tennis can put a lot of stress or repetitive activity on one's limbs. It is important to know if the activity was something performed prior to lymphedema. If the patient wants to resume the activity in order to exercise, have fun, and to have good quality of life, a sports fitness program can be instituted. This should be performed under medical guidance. In a sports fitness program, the muscles used in the sport are progressively strengthened so that the sport can be resumed. Patients must use caution as they return to a sport.

One of the most important things that can be done to decrease the risk of lymphedema is to keep weight at a good level. Those individuals with whom I have worked who have had lymphedema typically see a marked reduction of swelling in conjunction with weight loss. My students who are successful in losing weight have the most success in lymphedema control. Proper nutrition is important and decrease salt intake. Evidence suggests numerous benefits of exercise: improved fitness level, physical performance, quality of life, and less depression and fatigue. Exercise is part of a healthy lifestyle and will help in weight control and emotional health. There are exercise programs that are targeted at cancer survivors but not all of them will meet the needs of someone at risk for lymphedema. My goal is for cancer survivors to participate in individually structured and group exercise programs at all cancer centers or facilities close to their homes.

Exercise Tips from "10 to Thrive"

Carol Michaels wrote "Survivorship Care: Exercising and Health," published in "10 to Thrive" - an easy-to-navigate eBook of top 10 lists dealing with 10 different areas of a young adult survivor's life. The content in the eBook is supplied by experts, leaders and organizations in the cancer community.

At least 20 observational studies have shown that physically active cancer survivors have a lower risk of cancer recurrences and improved survival compared with those who are inactive, according to the newly released American Cancer Society 2012 Nutrition and Physical Activity Guidelines for Cancer Survivors.[1]

However, Dr. Demark-Winfried, associate director for cancer prevention and control at the University of Alabama at Birmingham, notes, "We know that after a first diagnosis of a potentially life-threatening cancer, many cancer survivors are primed to re-evaluate lifestyle behaviors; however, the data are beginning to accrue that this often is a short-term change, and without reinforcement, they tend to drift back to previous lifestyle habits the farther they are from diagnosis".[2]

What often gets in the way between survivors knowing they "should" exercise and actually doing it is an incorrect assumption. I have observed that many people assume that exercise has to be intense and high impact. An effective exercise program for cancer survivors, however, will start gently with slow progression. A good exercise program should take into account:

    i.   what exercises you already do,

    ii.   your limits,

    iii.   what you can do now and

    iv.   it should meet your interest and needs.

There are so many types of cancers, treatments and late term side effects and each one can affect survivors in different ways. It is important, therefore, to work with an exercise specialist or even possibly a physical therapist in order to develop the correct program for each unique situation. Check with your primary physician or other specialists tracking your survivorship care for recommendations to qualified exercise providers.

151

1. Getting Started

It is never too soon or too late to implement an exercise program. Just be sure you have received clearance from your doctor. A cancer exercise specialist can recommend a program that fits your unique needs. One of the best ways to find an exercise specialist is by contacting the American College of Sports Medicine-ACSM. Use the following link to find a specialist in your area: http://members.acsm.org.

Your exercise program will depend on your level of fitness prior to diagnosis, the type of cancer you had and the nature of your treatment. Before beginning any exercise program, it is important that your specialist conduct a full fitness assessment so that the exercise program will take into account your unique health issues and treatments. You should be aware of balance problems, weakness, and do not exercise if you become dizzy, anemic, or have an irregular heartbeat.

Deep breathing is a good way to begin each session. You can do this while lying down. Breathe in through the nose for 5 seconds and out of the mouth for 5 seconds. On the exhale press your navel to your spine. Deep breathing is a great way to calm the nerves and has a calming effect. If you have or are at risk for lymphedema, deep breathing can aid lymphatic flow. Lymphedema is an accumulation of lymphatic fluid, which can cause swelling. It can develop at any time so use judgment when exercising. A lymphedema specialist, physical therapist or cancer exercise specialist can review this with you. http://lymphnet.org is a great source of information on this topic.

2. Aerobic Exercises

Aerobic exercise gets the heart rate up and includes activity like walking, biking and running. The American cancer Society recommends "Adults should get at least 150 minutes of moderate intensity or 75 minutes of vigorous intensity activity each week (or a combination of these), preferably spread throughout the week."

Your conditioning at the time you start exercising will govern your program. For those of you who have not done any exercise, walking is a good start. You should have a goal of building it up to at least 30 to 60 minutes almost daily. You can do it all at once or break it up in small amounts done throughout the day. Pay attention to your heart rate, breathing and muscle fatigue. It may be counter intuitive but if you suffer from fatigue, exercise may help. So set up a routine for when you have more energy and it is not necessary to go past moderate intensity.

Aerobic exercise is a good way to burn calories to keep your weight under control. Being over weight will exacerbate other medical conditions a cancer survivor may have. Exercise may also reduce the risk of a cancer recurrence. Evidence that exercise can reduce the risk of dying of cancer is accumulating; the benefits of exercise to your lungs, heart and other organs are established. There is growing evidence that the amount of time spent sitting is important, regardless of your activity level. Our lifestyle is causing us to be less active. Too many of us sit in front of a computer or TV for hours at a time. So try to get up and walk around or stretch every half hour.

In a group of 3000 women with breast cancer, the ones who exercised (3mph walking) about 30 minutes/day, 5 days per week had 50% greater survival than those who weren't as active.[3]

3. Posture and Balance

Surgery and radiation can result in muscle tightness, which causes poor posture. Poor posture is one of the reasons some survivors have aches and pains and it can lead to orthopedic issues. Some of the chemotherapies can affect balance and cause neuropathy. Begin with neck, shoulder and upper back stretches. Simple exercise like walking on a straight line like a tightrope and calf raises can improve balance. The American Cancer Society's web site www.cancer.org is a good place to start your search for information.

4. Flexibility

Lack of flexibility is another important concern. Survivors need to learn appropriate stretches and continue to perform them long after surgery and treatments are finished. Surgery and treatments often result in a decrease in range of motion. Ideally, you should begin a stretching program to stay flexible and maintain flexibility as soon as you can. If you did not start right after treatment, you should not use that as an excuse not to start now. You can start a stretching program at any time and improve your flexibility. Scar tissue will continue to form and must be stretched regularly to prevent adhesions. Survivors find that they need to continue to stretch long after their surgery and treatments. A good way to start is to go to www.recoveryfitness.net where you can find a DVD, which covers essential stretches to regain your flexibility.

5. Strength Training

Strength training increases muscle mass. It can be performed with weights, bands, machines, or your own body weight. Some treatments can cause sarcopenia, which is a change in the fat:muscle ratio. Strength training is important because it can increase your muscle mass and decrease fat.

Overweight women have a higher risk of recurrence compared to women who maintain a health weight. Estrogen receptor positive breast cancer is fed by estrogen, which thrives in fat. Dr. Jennifer Ligibel, a medical oncologist at the Dana Farber Cancer Center found that BMI was related to survival. The National Cancer Institute's November 2011 bulletin states "Obesity has been linked with increase risk of recurrence and death in several cancers. For example recent findings from the California Teachers Study showed that being obese at the time of study entry was associated with a substantial increase in the risk of dying from breast cancer in several subgroups, including women who have been treated for estrogen receptor positive breast cancer."

Strength training can also help decrease the risk of osteoporosis, which can be an issue after chemotherapy. Strength training will not only increase your muscle mass, it will also help to strengthen your bones. Reconstructive surgeries usually require special strength training exercise programs.

6. Overall Health Benefit

An exercise program will improve your overall health. Exercise improves your chances of surviving cancer and reduces many long-term late side effects of the treatments. It can help your heart, bones, and decrease your risk of diabetes. Starting an exercise program can be a challenge - even for healthy people. Just think of all the benefits to exercise. It can improve the chance of being there for your children and grandchildren. You will also be a healthy lifestyle role model for your family. It will increase your energy and concentration so that you can perform better at work. Exercise will improve your quality of life. It will enable you to participate in the sports and activities that you enjoy and you will feel better physically and emotionally.

7. Weight Control

Exercise will help you control your weight. Many people actually wind up gaining weight from the cancer treatments. This is a health concern for all survivors, however it can be particularly harmful for breast cancer patients with estrogen positive cancers. Exercise will help you lose weight and rebuild muscle to increase metabolism. For those of you who need to gain weight, exercise can help increase your appetite. Gastro-intestinal cancers and head and neck cancer can cause loss of muscle mass and weight loss.

Cancer can also take a toll on how you feel about your body. A lot of the surgeries and therapies required to treat a cancer can alter the body and make one feel badly about their body. Exercise makes you fitter, which improves body image. When you start to see the benefits of exercise it serves as positive reinforcement. Write down all the reasons to start a program: less fatigue, better mood, improved energy, feel better, etc. Scheduling your exercise in the morning and make that your priority before you start your day is a strategy that works for many of my clients. If you leave it for later in the day something might come up to interfere with your program. A good approach is to have an exercise friend. You will both reinforce each other and you will be accountable to each other.

8. Reduce Stress

Exercise can decrease stress, anxiety, and depression. Regular exercise has a powerful effect on one's mood by releasing pain-relieving endorphins. Always start slowly and listen to your body eventually increasing the frequency, length, and intensity of your program. Exercise training is emerging as a therapy to the negative psychological side effects associated with cancer. Make sure your exercise program is fun. Exercising with friends builds a social camaraderie. Group exercise classes provide friendship and support and motivate you to stick to a program.

9. Commitment to Start

Starting an exercise program is difficult, but so rewarding. All types of moderate exercise are beneficial. Think about the activities or sports that you enjoy and do them. Do you like to walk, ride a bicycle, or dance? If so, you can build your exercise program around the activity you find enjoyable. Notice if you start making excuses for not exercising.

We often use excuses to hide our fear of failure. They then become a barrier to achieving our goals. Women with breast cancer or survivors who are uncomfortable with the physical changes caused by cancer or treatment, may have unique concerns about their appearance and may be uncomfortable when changing in a locker room or wearing certain kinds of workout gear or bathing suits. If you need a private changing area, request one. Choose clothing you feel physically and mentally comfortable wearing. Thanks to the Internet, there are many sites to help you find what you need. Self-advocacy is an important part of empowering yourself in survivorship. Rely on your inner strength to exceed self-imposed limitations. A fear of believing that you won't achieve goals can prevent you from trying.

10. Maintaining Your Exercise Program

How can you stick with your exercise program? It is a good idea to set goals. Some people derive great satisfaction in setting and then achieving goals. You can record your daily progress. This can be done with charts and graphs to record your progress and reward achievements. You will feel good about yourself when you achieve your goals. Cancer survivors can show tremendous progress when participating in a consistent well-designed exercise program. You should keep in mind that just like everyone else, you will have good and bad days so you should be able to adapt. Keep as active as possible, be safe and have fun.

There is a very important message for cancer survivors and patients - stay active. Research has shown physical and emotional improvement after participation in exercise. The American Cancer Society's April 2013 newsletter states "Among breast cancer survivors, a recent analysis shows that getting exercise after diagnosis was associated with a 34% lowered risk of breast cancer death, a 41% lower risk of dying from all causes, and a 24% lowered risk of breast cancer recurrence. Among colon cancer, studies suggest exercise cuts death from colon cancer and all causes, and cuts the risk of the cancer coming back by up to 50%.

---

[1] Rock, C. L., Doyle, C., Demark - Wahnefried, W., Meyerhardt, J., Courneya, K. S., Schwartz, A. L., Bandera, E. V., Hamilton, K. K., Grant, B., McCullough, M., Byers, T. and Gansler, T. (2012), Nutrition and physical activity guidelines for cancer survivors. CA: A Cancer Journal for Clinicians, 62: 242–274. doi: 10.3322/caac.21142
http://onlinelibrary.wiley.com/doi/10.3322/caac.21142/abstract

[2] Encouraging Lifestyle Modifications, Personalizing Surveillance Strategies Improves Risk of Second Cancer , ASCO Daily News,
http://chicago2012.asco.org/ASCODailyNews/Survivorprevention.aspx

[3] Holmes MD, Chen WY, Feskanich D, Kroenke CH, Colditz GA. Physical Activity and Survival After Breast Cancer Diagnosis. *JAMA*. 2005;293 (20):2479-2486. doi:10.1001/jama.293.20.2479.

Health Needs of Low Income Communities

My community involvement inspired me to focus my goals on expanding health education, exercise, and achieving healthy productive lifestyles for my clients in suburban and urban communities.

I am currently an officer and a trustee of the Musical Instrument Donation Program. This charity collects musical instruments and distributes them to those that cannot afford to buy or rent one. One significant aspect of the process is that I visit schools and meet residents and teachers in low-income communities. My work for this charity opened my eyes to the health needs of low-income communities. Many residents suffer from chronic conditions and do not have health insurance or the ability to pay for rehabilitation. Our musical instrument charity made me aware of the fitness and health services that were needed in certain areas. After meeting so many people in need while delivering instruments, I decided something needed to be done.

I met with several people at the Cancer Center of Newark Beth Israel who were very encouraging and receptive. I donated my time and we established a pilot program for cancer patients. This consisted of free exercise classes at the Cancer Center of Newark Beth Israel for one year. During the year, we monitored various fitness markers. We took range of motion measurements and recorded strength levels for each participant. Arm measurements were also taken to monitor for lymphedema. The results of the one-year program were compiled and they were terrific: increased range of motion, increased strength, decrease in lymphedema and emotional improvement.

Recovery Fitness® has a broad impact in a number of communities. I educate cancer survivors about the importance of exercise and healthy lifestyles. The results from the Recovery Fitness® program have been excellent in both urban and suburban communities. These classes enable survivors with limited financial means to improve their health and become active productive members of their community. Our classes not only help the participants heal physically, but also help to restore their self esteem. They are empowered to go back to their jobs and families and take charge of their lives.

About the Authors

Carol Michaels is the founder and creator of Recovery Fitness®, an exercise program designed to help cancer patients recover from surgery and treatments. She owns and operates Recovery Fitness and Carol Michaels Fitness in Short Hills, New Jersey and is a trailblazer in the area of cancer exercise. She has worked with physicians and other health professionals to develop her program, which is currently offered 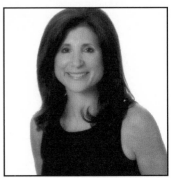 at her studio, two hospitals and two community centers. She understands the needs of cancer survivors and developed a practical program to help them reach their goals.

Carol is a Cancer Exercise Specialist and consultant and has been a fitness professional for more than 17 years. She received her degree from the Wharton School of the University of Pennsylvania and is certified by the Cancer Exercise Training Institute, American Council on Exercise, American College of Sports Medicine (ACSM), and is a member of ACSM and IDEA Health and Fitness Association.

Carol is a speaker for corporate wellness programs, fundraisers, and community events on fitness and health issues. She is on the advisory board of Living Beyond Breast Cancer, and is an ambassador for HERA Women's Cancer Foundation. She has recently held workshops for: The American Cancer Society, Gilda's Club, FORCE, Atlantic Healthy Lifestyles, Pathways, St. Barnabas Hospital, and Morristown Medical Center.

Carol has appeared on health-related television programs. She authored a chapter in the e-book *Ten to Thrive*. She was a columnist for *PFP Magazine*, and has written for The American Academy of Health and Fitness, The National Lymphedema Network, 4wholeness.com™, and the Pink Paper.

The American Council on Exercise and Life Fitness recognized her as a Trainer to Watch in 2011. Personal Fitness Professional honored her as the 2012 PFP Trainer of the Year. Carol developed and produced two DVDs called Recovery Fitness Cancer Exercise-Simple Stretches and Recovery Fitness-Strength Training. Both DVDs can be found on her websites: www.recoveryfitness.net. and www.carolmichaelsfitness.com.

Maria Drozda earned a Bachelor of Arts degree in Dance and a Master of Business Administration from the State University of New York at Buffalo (UB). After serving as a teaching assistant in UB's Department of Theater and Dance, she choreographed and performed with musical theater companies, dance companies and dance schools in Buffalo, NY; Tracy, CA; and Hampton, VA.

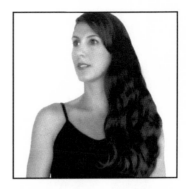

Maria gained business experience across a broad range of sectors including educational institutions, private industry, a government research lab, and non-profit organizations. Taking on varied roles, she contributed to the success of her employers through leadership development and succession planning, internal communications and change management, recruiting and staffing, business analysis, conference and event planning, and print and web publication.

When her children were born, Maria developed a passion for fitness for mothers of young children and became an American Council on Exercise (ACE) certified group fitness instructor with specialty certification in pre-natal and post-natal fitness. She taught fitness classes for new and expecting mothers via the Stroller Strides® franchises in Tracy, CA and Hampton, VA, and created her own stroller-based fitness program in Indianapolis, IN. These programs have empowered mothers to regain and maintain their health and fitness levels as well as become healthy role models for their children.

Maria enjoys consulting and freelance writing. She was thrilled to be invited to partner with Carol Michaels in the writing of this book, and hopes that it will help cancer survivors achieve excellent physical comfort and fitness to enjoy the activities they love.